Treatment of Neurological Disorders with Intravenous Immunoglobulins

Edited by
GÉRARD SAID MD
PROFESSOR AND CHAIRMAN
SERVICE DE NEUROLOGIE
CHU DE BICÊTRE
UNIVERSITÉ PARIS-SUD
PARIS

MARTIN DUNITZ

© Martin Dunitz 2000

First published in the United Kingdom in 2000 by:
Martin Dunitz Ltd
The Livery House
7–9 Pratt Street
London NW1 0AE

Tel: +44 (0)207 482 2202
Fax: +44 (0)207 267 0159
E-mail: info@mdunitz.globalnet.co.uk
Website: http://www.dunitz.co.uk

All rights reserved. No part of this publication may be reproduced, stored in a retrieval system or transmitted, in any form or by any means, without the prior permission of the publisher or in accordance with the provisions of the Copyright Act 1988.

A CIP record for this book is available from the British Library

ISBN 1-85317-758-X

Distributed in the United States by:
Blackwell Science Inc
Commerce Place, 350 Main Street
Malden MA 02148, USA
Tel: 1 800 215 1000

Distributed in Canada by:
Login Brothers Book Company
324 Salteaux Crescent
Winnipeg, Manitoba R3J 3T2
Canada
Tel: 1 204 224 4068

Distributed in Brazil by:
Ernesto Reichmann Distribuidora de Livros, Ltda
Rua Coronel Marques 335, Tatuape 03440-000
Sao Paulo
Brazil

Composition by Wearset, Boldon, Tyne and Wear
Printed and bound in Italy

Contents

Contributors   *v*
Preface   *vii*

1. **Intravenous immunoglobulins: impact on effector mechanisms in autoimmune neurological disorders**   *1*
   Hans-Peter Hartung, Bernd C Kieseier, Ralf Gold and Juan J Archelos

2. **Multifocal neuropathies**   *19*
   Richard A Lewis

3. **Chronic inflammatory demyelinating polyneuropathy**   *43*
   Pieter A van Doorn

4. **Prognostic factors in chronic inflammatory demyelinating polyneuropathy**   *57*
   Gérard Said

5. **Inflammatory myopathies**   *67*
   Marinos C Dalakas

6. **Guillain–Barré syndrome**   *83*
   David R Cornblath

7. **Myasthenia gravis and the Lambert–Eaton myasthenic syndrome**   *93*
   John Newsom-Davis

8	**Relapsing–remitting multiple sclerosis**	**103**
	Frans Fazekas	
9	**Neuro-Behçet syndrome**	**115**
	Aksel Siva and Ayşe Altıntaş	
10	**West syndrome and Lennox–Gastaut syndrome**	**127**
	Willy O Renier	
11	**Intravenous immunoglobulins: preparation, safety and clinical use**	**135**
	Rainer H Böger and Stefanie M Bode-Böger	
12	**Safety and tolerability of intravenous immunoglobulins**	**181**
	Turf D Martin	

Contributors

Ayşe Altıntaş MD
Associate Professor of Neurology, Istanbul University, Cerrahpaşa School of Medicine, Istanbul, Turkey.

Juan J Archelos
Klinische Abteilung für Allgemeine Neurologie, Universitätsklinik für Neurologie, Landeskrankenhaus–Universitätsklinikum Graz, Karl-Franzens-Universität, Graz, Austria.

Stefanie M Bode-Böger MD
Assistant Professor of Clinical Pharmacology, Institute of Clinical Pharmacology, Medical School, Hannover, Germany.

Rainer H Böger MD
Assistant Professor of Clinical Pharmacology, Institute of Clinical Pharmacology, Medical School, Hannover, Germany.

David R Cornblath MD
Professor, Department of Neurology, Johns Hopkins University School of Medicine, Baltimore MD, USA.

Marinos C Dalakas MD
Chief, Neuromuscular Diseases Section, National Institute of Neurological Disorders and Stroke, National Institutes of Health, Bethesda MD, USA.

Franz Fazekas MD
Department of Neurology and MRI Center, Karl-Franzens University, Graz, Austria.

Ralf Gold
Klinische Abteilung für Allgemeine Neurologie, Universitätsklinik für Neurologie, Landeskrankenhaus–Universitätsklinikum Graz, Karl-Franzens-Universität, Graz, Austria.

Hans-Peter Hartung MD
Professor and Head, Klinische Abteilung für Allgemeine Neurologie, Universitätsklinik für Neurologie, Landeskrankenhaus–Universitätsklinikum Graz, Karl-Franzens-Universität, Graz, Austria.

Bernd C Kieseier MD
Universitätsklinik für Neurologie, Julius-Maximilians-Universitäts Würzburg, Germany

Richard A Lewis MD
Department of Neurology, Wayne State University School of Medicine, Detroit MI, USA.

Turf D Martin
Octapharma AG, Lachen, Switzerland.

John Newsom-Davis MD FRCP FRS
Professor Emeritus, Department of Clinical Neurology, University of Oxford, Radcliffe Infirmary, Oxford, UK.

Willy O Renier MD PhD
Associate Professor of Epilepsy, University Hospital of Nijmegen, Nijmegen, The Netherlands.

Gérard Said MD
Professor and Chairman, Service de Neurologie, Centre Hospitalier Universitaire de Bicêtre, Université Paris-Sud, Le Kremlin Bicêtre, Paris, France.

Aksel Siva MD
Professor of Neurology, Istanbul University, Cerrahpaşa School of Medicine, Istanbul, Turkey.

Pieter A van Doorn MD
Neurologist, Department of Neurology, University Hospital Rotterdam, Rotterdam, The Netherlands.

Preface

The last decade has seen the introduction of intravenous immunoglobulin as a new treatment regimen in the treatment of peripheral nerve diseases and a subset of central nerve diseases. While the superior benefit of intravenous immunoglobulin has yet to be established in many of these disease states, many patients have benefited from a significant improvement in their clinical conditions and quality of life. The Committee of Proprietary Medicinal Products of the European Union has recently recommended that Guillain-Barré syndrome be added as a full indication for intravenous immunoglobulins. This book is broadly based on a symposium held at the 1998 European Neurological Society annual meeting in Nice, France. It provides a current view of the status of intravenous immunoglobulin in the treatment of peripheral and central nerve diseases. We hope that you find it valuable in understanding the current and future role of intravenous immunoglobulin in the clinical treatment of these diseases which will result in continued patient recovery from these debilitating conditions.

Turf D Martin
International Business Manager
Immunology Division
Octapharma AG
Lachen, Switzerland
June 2000

Intravenous immunoglobulins: impact on effector mechanisms in autoimmune neurological disorders

Hans-Peter Hartung, Bernd C Kieseier, Ralf Gold and Juan J Archelos

> ADCC: antibody-dependent cellular cytotoxicity; CIDP: chronic inflammatory demyelinating polyradiculoneuropathy; EAE: experimental allergic encephalomyelitis; EAN: experimental autoimmune neuritis; Fab: fragment, antigen-binding; Fc: fragment, crystallizable; GBS: Guillain–Barré syndrome; HLA: human leukocyte antigens; IFN: interferon; Ig: immunoglobulin; IL: interleukin; IVIG: intravenous immunoglobulin; LEMS: Lambert–Eaton myasthenic syndrome; LFA: lymphocyte function-associated antigen; LT: lymphotoxin; MAC: membrane attack complex; MHC: major histocompatibility complex; MS; multiple sclerosis; TCR: T-cell receptor; TGF: transforming growth factor; TNF: tumour necrosis factor

Introduction

Since the fortuitous discovery of high-dose intravenous immunoglobulin (IVIG) as an effective treatment for idiopathic thrombocytopenic purpura in the late 1970s, an ever-growing number of diseases considered to be autoimmune in nature have been shown to respond to such therapy. There is now direct evidence, based on controlled trials as well as circumstantial, that IVIG is (partially) effective in Guillain–Barré syndrome, chronic inflammatory demyelinating polyradiculoneuropathy (CIDP), paraproteinaemic neuropathies, myasthenia gravis, Lambert–Eaton myasthenic syndrome (LEMS), dermatomyositis and multiple sclerosis (MS).[1–3] All these diseases affecting the neuraxis at different levels are considered to result from aberrant T-cellular and/or humoral immune responses.

Composition of commercially available IVIG

Commercial IVIG batches are derived from human plasma of 2000–5000 donors by Cohn's process, i.e. cold ethanol fractionation. Purification is achieved through enzymatic treatment at low pH, fractionation and chromatography. In most preparations, more than 95% is immunoglobulin G (IgG), less than 2.5% IgA. IgG1 makes up 55–70%, IgG2 0–6% and IgG4 0–2.5%. IVIG contains 40% dimers and 60% monomers (*Fig. 1.1*).[4]

The IgG molecule

An antibody molecule of IgG consists of four polypeptide chains. There are two light chains (L) and two heavy chains (H). The L chain has a variable (V) fragment with 108–111 amino acid residues and a constant (C) component of about 105 residues (*Fig. 1.2*). In an H chain, the V domain is composed of the products of three genes, V_H, D and J_H. Three C domains each encoded by a single gene (C_H1, C_H2, C_H3) are connected to the

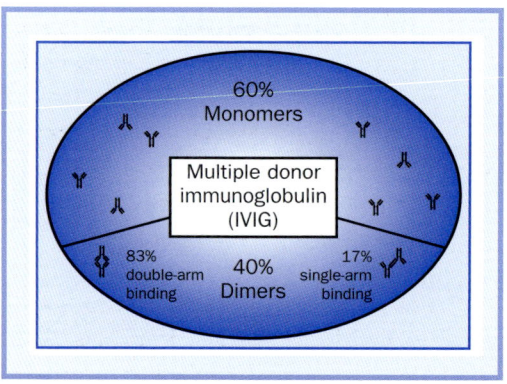

Figure 1.1
Commercial IVIG preparations. Individual batches are derived from 2000–5000 donors. The fractionation process results in the presence of 60% monomers and 40% dimers of which 83% are double-arm binding and 17% single-arm binding.

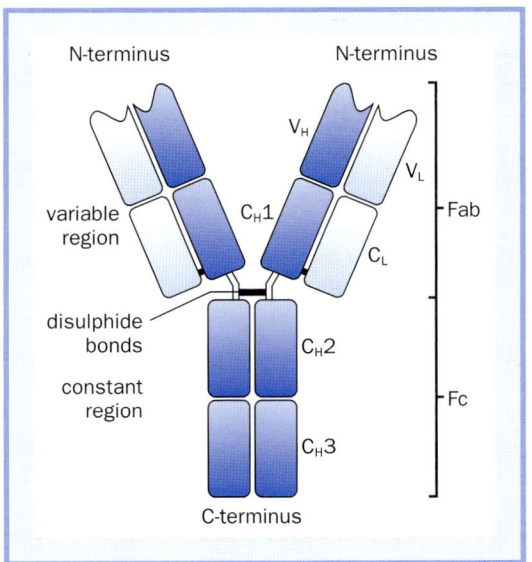

Figure 1.2
Basic structure of the IgG molecule.

V_H domain. One L and one H chain are normally covalently linked by a disulphide bond. V_L and V_H domains are noncovalently linked to form a variable fragment region, the tip of which forms the binding site for antigen. V and C pairs constitute the Fab portion (fragment, antigen binding) (*Fig. 1.2*).

The functions of immunoglobulins, including IgG, are manifold but all essentially serve to neutralize foreign antigens (*Table 1.1*). An enormous degree of molecular flexibility allows recognition of a myriad of antigens. The principal effector functions mediated by antibodies are complement activation, phagocytosis and antibody-dependent cellular cytotoxicity (*Fig. 1.3*). The classical pathway of complement is triggered by the interaction of complement component C1q with IgG. IgG3 and IgG1 efficiently activate human complement. The binding site for C1q is located on the final beta strand of the C_H2 domain.

Immunoglobulin G binds to Fc receptors on various human leukocytes and these receptors come in three classes: FcRγI, FcRγII, FcRγIII. The first, also termed CD64, is expressed on monocytes, macrophages, dendritic cells and stimulated neutrophils. FcRγII, also referred to as CD32, is broadly expressed on most leukocytes and

Table 1.1
Possible mechanisms of IVIG action*

Possible mechanism of IVIG action	Literature*	Comment
Antiidiotypic antibodies	Jayne et al 1999; Jefferis 1993; Ronda et al 1994	Antiidiotype antibodies against autoantibodies can bind these and neutralize them. There are some suggestions that this mechanism could be of importance in Guillain–Barré syndrome
Inhibition of antibody production of B cells	Bijsterbosch and Klaus 1985; Kondo et al 1991;	Antiidiotypes can also bind on membrane-bound antibodies on the surface of B cells and shut down the immunoglobulin production
Inhibition of CD5-positive cells	Vassilev et al 1993	CD5 is expressed on the majority of T cells and a subset of B cells that synthesize low-affinity polyreactive autoantibodies. Antibodies against CD5 have been shown to be contained in IVIG
Blockage of Fc receptors	Heyman 1990	Intact IgG can bind with its constant region to Fc receptors of cells of the reticuloendothelial system. This mechanism seems to be important in idiopathic thrombocytopenic purpura (Debre et al 1993)
Modulation of T-cell activation via soluble molecules	Grosse-Wilde et al 1992; Blasczyk et al 1993; Perosa et al 1995	Soluble CD4, CD8 and MHC molecules contained in IVIG can act as antagonists of the T-cell receptor and thus block activation
Antiidiotypic effect on T-cell receptors	Marchalonis et al 1992	Antibodies against the T-cell receptor β-chain can block T-cell activation. They were shown to be present in sera from healthy individuals
Enhancement of CD8-positive suppressor T-cell function	Delfraissy et al 1985; Leung et al 1987; Ballow et al 1989	Increased numbers of CD8-positive suppressor cells and increased suppressor T-cell function was noted after IVIG treatment
Neutralization of superantigens	Takei et al 1993	Neutralizing antibodies to bacterial or viral superantigens, which may activate T cells nonspecifically, have been shown to be present in IVIG

Table 1.1
Continued

Possible mechanism of IVIG action	Literature*	Comment
Neutralization of toxins and pathogens	Masson 1993	Direct binding of antigens that initiate or perpetuate the autoimmune reaction
Modulation of cytokine production by immune cells	Andersson et al 1993; Klaesson et al 1993; Skansen-Saphir et al 1994; Ruiz de Souza et al 1995	Modulation of expression of various cytokines was shown in vitro after addition of IVIG to lymphocyte cultures. Reduction of IL-1 production was demonstrated in Kawasaki syndrome (Leung et al 1989). Decreased TNFα production was suggested to be responsible for the therapeutic effect of IVIG in experimental allergic encephalomyelitis, an animal model resembling multiple sclerosis (Achiron et al 1994)
Direct binding of cytokines	Svenson et al 1993; Okitsu-Negishi et al 1994; Ros et al 1995	Binding antibodies against IL-1, IL-6, IFNα and INFβ were shown to be present in IVIG preparations
Inhibition of complement-mediated effects	Basta et al 1989; Frank et al 1992	IgG can bind complement and thus inhibit the damage following complement activation. Decrease of C3c was noted in IVIG-treated patients with myasthenia (Kamolvarin et al), and deposition of activated complement was blocked in dermatomyositis (Basta and Dalakas 1994)
Increase of Ig catabolism	Masson 1993	The catabolic rate of immunoglobulins increases with higher serum concentrations and thus the half-life of autoantibodies is decreased

*For references see Stangel et al 1998.[2]

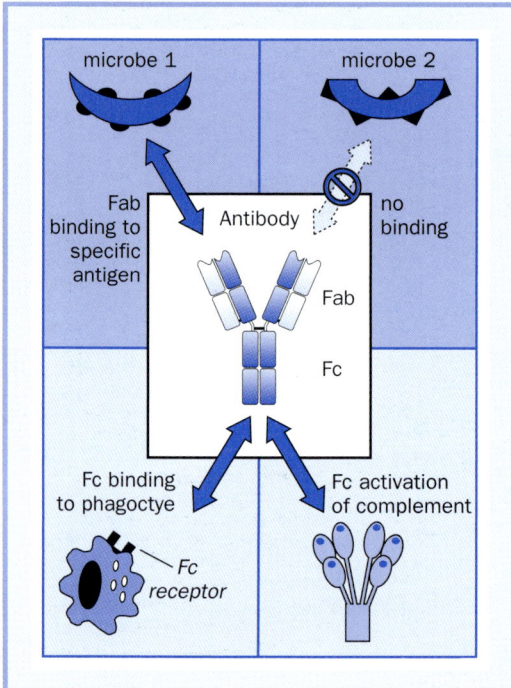

Figure 1.3
Basic functions of the IgG molecule. The essential task of antibodies including IgG is elimination of invading foreign antigens. This is achieved in multiple ways and involves direct recognition through the Fab fragment or the triggering of effector mechanisms through the Fc portion of the molecule.

FcRγIII (CD16) can be detected on macrophages, natural killer cells and subsets of T cells.

A number of functionally relevant sites can be differentiated on an antibody molecule (*Fig. 1.4*).

Suppression of antibody production

One of the mechanisms first suggested to be responsible for IVIG effects is downregulation of the production of antibodies including autoantibodies by B lymphocytes. IgG via its Fc fragment binds to corresponding cellular receptors. Cross-linking of neighbouring Fc receptors to which IgG molecules are attached delivers a negative signal to the B cell that reduces its synthesis of immunoglobulins (*Fig. 1.5*).[5–7]

Preparations of IVIG have also been shown to contain antibodies to CD5 molecules.[8] These are expressed on the surface of a particular subset of B cells that generate

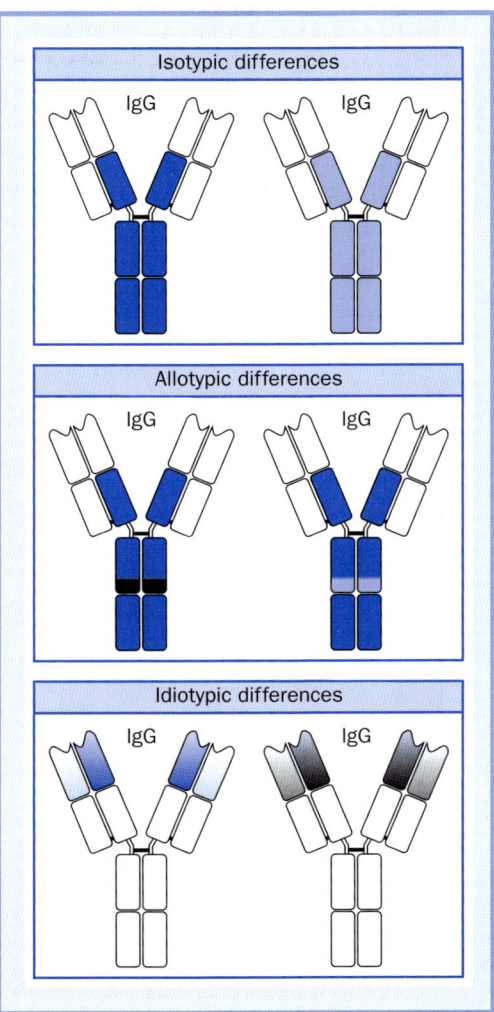

Figure 1.4
IgG: partial differentiation. Immunoglobulin isotypes are responsible for the biological effector functions of antibody molecules. Heavy-chain isotypes determine the subclass of immunoglobulins (IgA, IgG, IgD, IgG, IgM). IgG has four subclasses: IgG1–IgG4. IgG antibodies are the predominant isotype of the secondary antibody response.

Allotypes reflect the existence of two or more variants of a given gene encoding for immunoglobulins. The allotype of an Ig molecule is recognized by the expression of the unique epitope (referred to as the allotope) and is designated by a capital letter representing the heavy-chain, isotype or light-chain type. There is some evidence that antibody molecules of the same isotype but different allotypes may differ in their potential to activate effector mechanisms.

The unique tertiary structure of the antigen binding site of an antigen-specific receptor is referred to as the idiotype. When antigen-specific antibodies are in turn used as antigens, immune responses occur to the idiotypic regions of the molecules. Such responses are called antiidiotypic and may serve an important role in maintaining immune homeostasis.

low-affinity, high-avidity polyreactive 'natural' autoantibodies.[9–11] Some of the glycolipid antibodies described in immune-mediated neuropathies may be part of this natural autoantibody repertoire (*Fig. 1.6*).[12,13]

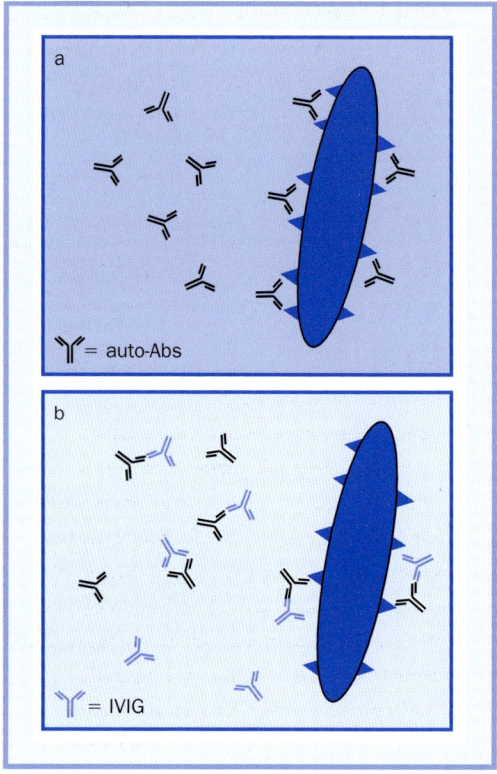

Figure 1.5
Inhibition of antibody production. Binding of antibody to the B cell surface delivers a negative signal resulting in downregulation of antibody production including synthesis of autoantibodies by B lymphocytes.

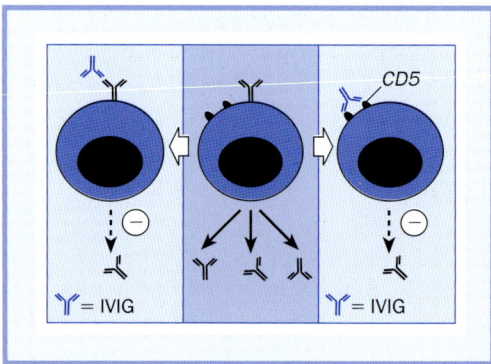

Figure 1.6
Downregulation of the synthesis of natural autoantibodies. A specific subset of B cells identifiable by the surface expression of the CD5 antigen releases antibodies of low affinity but high avidity. These antibodies form part of a natural repertoire available to any individual. IVIG preparations have been shown to contain antibodies to CD5 and may thereby potentially downregulate the production of pathogenic autoantibodies.

Neutralization of autoantibodies

Preparations of IVIG can be considered to represent the collective immunological memory of some 2000–5000 individuals. They contain 'antiidiotypic' antibodies that by binding to and neutralizing pathogenic autoantibodies maintain immune homeostasis in an idiotype–antiidiotype network.[9,10,14–17] Such a mechanism has been proposed to be at work in CIDP and GM1-antibody-mediated neuropathies as well as in LEMS and myasthenia gravis.[13,15,18–20]

Neutralization of complement-mediated effects

Antibodies can cause tissue damage through activation of the complement system with subsequent release of proinflammatory peptides such as C3a and C5a, phagocytosis-promoting factors such as C3b and the assembly of the membrane attack complex (MAC) made up of the terminal complement components C5b-9. MAC can permeabilize membranes, precipitating an influx of calcium that can in turn activate membrane-integral proteases. Insertion of MAC into myelin membranes may be a crucial effector mechanism of demyelination. IVIG apparently is capable of inhibiting cellular uptake of complement fragments C3 and C4, disrupting the formation and deposition of MAC.[21] Evidence is available to suggest that such a mechanism contributes to therapeutic efficacy in dermatomyositis, Guillain–Barré syndrome (GBS) and myasthenia gravis (*Fig. 1.7*).[22–26]

Interference with antibody-dependent cellular cytotoxicity

Macrophages are crucial effector cells in inflammatory demyelination both in the central nervous system (as in multiple sclerosis) and in peripheral nerves (as in GBS and CIDP). IVIG may bind to Fc receptors on macrophages and thereby modulate their affinity by either saturating, altering or downregulating them. Deactivation of a host of macrophage actions including phagocytosis and elaboration of an array of injurious molecules may be of key relevance to the therapeutic efficacy of IVIG in the above disorders. Saturation of Fc receptors or macrophages may also prevent binding of autoantibodies that could via their Fab fragment direct these phagocytic cells to their target antigen. Macrophages may thus be rendered unable to reach and damage target structures on neural tissues (*Figs 1.8, 1.9*).[18,25,27,28]

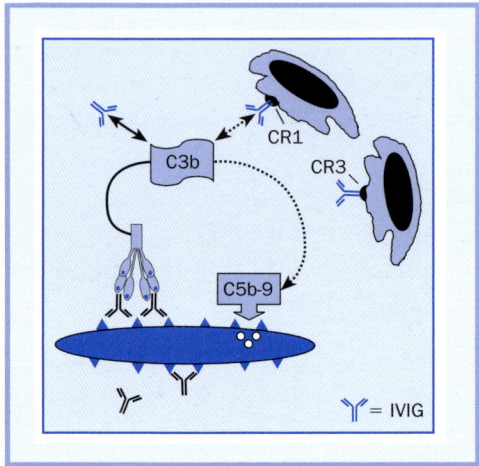

Figure 1.7
Neutralization of complement. IVIG may act by neutralizing complement, the major effector mechanism of the humoral immune system. By binding to C3b it may prevent the assembly of the C3 and C5 convertases and thereby block complement activation at an early step. Further, IVIG may block cellular receptors for activated complement and interfere with the formation of the terminal membrane attack complex (MAC, C5b–9).

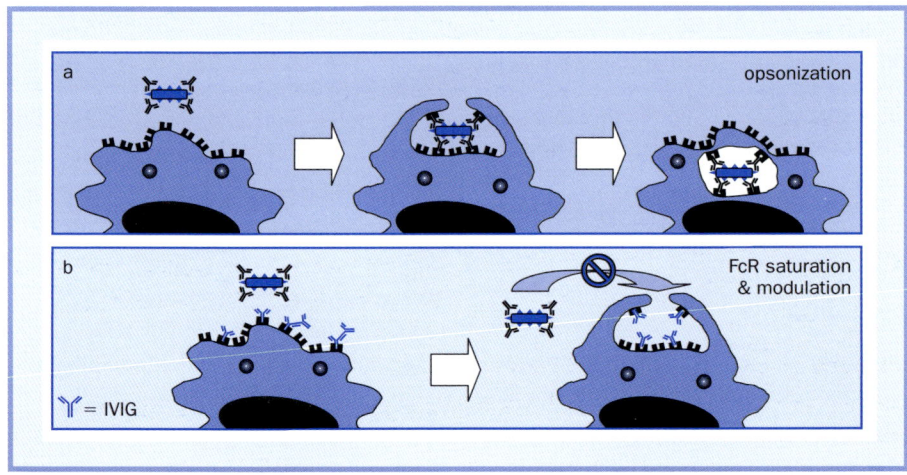

Figure 1.8
Modulation of Fc receptors. Fc receptors—amongst other functions—are important in triggering antibody-mediated cell activation. For example, foreign antigen covered by antibodies ('opsonized') is more readily taken up by macrophages. Autoantibodies binding to Fc receptors on macrophages may activate these to enhanced phagocytosis but also increased production of soluble noxious molecules. High-dose IVIG may saturate these surface receptors or change their affinity and therefore intervene with autoantibody-mediated cellular activation.

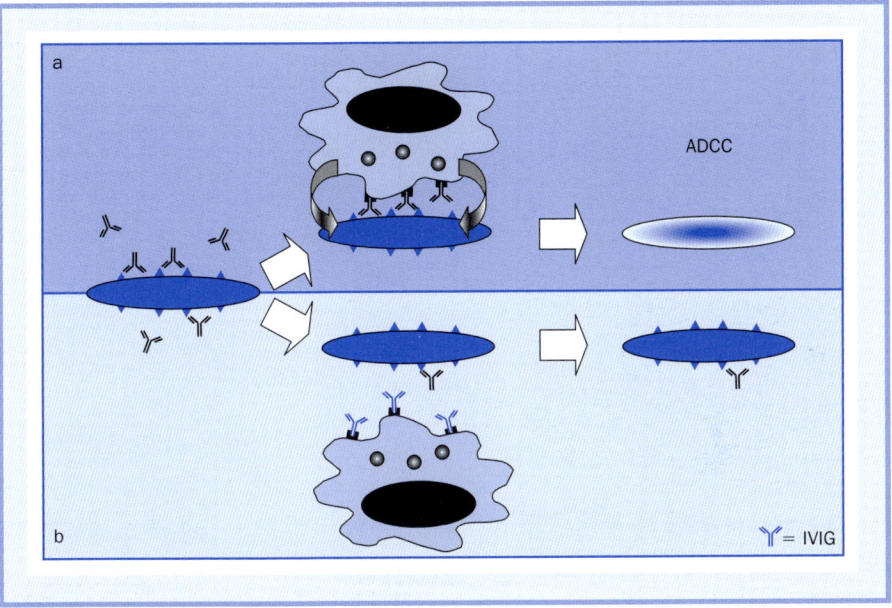

Figure 1.9
Inhibition of antibody-dependent cellular cytotoxicity by IVIG.

Acceleration of antibody metabolism

It has been observed that infusion of IVIG results in a shortened half-life of circulating immunoglobulin. Recently, a mechanism that may underlie the accelerated catabolism of endogenous IgG, including pathogenic IgG, has been proposed to involve binding to a protective receptor in endocytotic vesicles termed FcRn.[12] This binding prevents lysosomal degradation of IgG. Saturation of this FcRn by IVIG may result in the escape of endogenous IgG from these protective mechanisms.

Effects on T-cell activation

Preparations of IVIG have been documented to contain variable amounts of soluble CD4, CD8, HLA-I and HLA-II molecules that may interfere with the trimolecular interaction of T-cell receptor, autoantigenic epitopes and MHC recognition molecules, although this

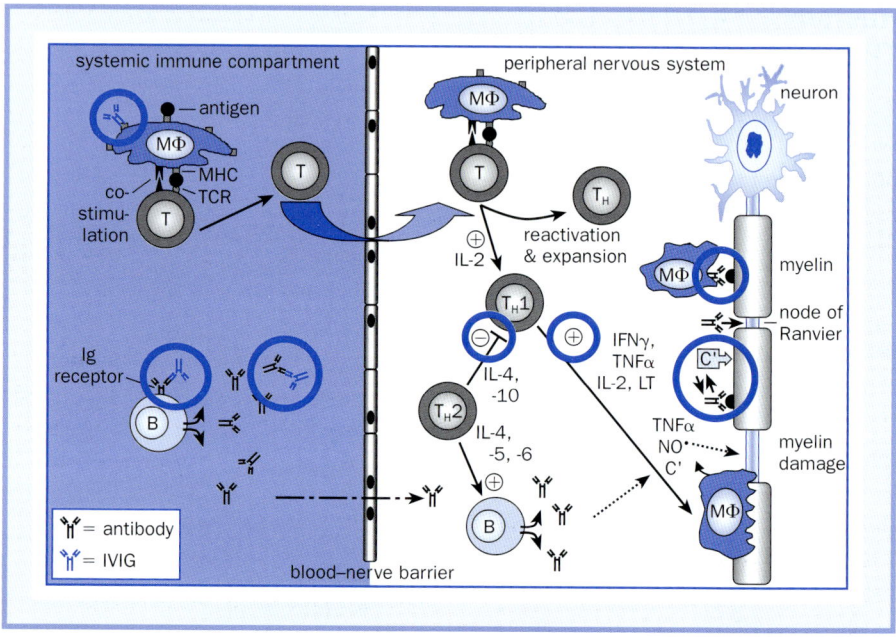

Figure 1.10
Synopsis: potential modes of action of IVIG in immune neuropathies. Immune neuropathies such as GBS and CIDP are thought to result from aberrant T and B cell responses launched to peripheral nerve antigens.[18,27] This synopsis summarizes the various pathogenic steps culminating in nerve damage and identifies potential sites of therapeutic intervention by IVIG (circles). In all likelihood, though, only some of the many potential actions may be clinically relevant.

notion has been challenged on methodological grounds.[2,29,30] This interference would blunt autoreactive T cells. Such an effect may also be brought about by antibodies shown to be present in IVIG that are capable of recognizing T-cell receptor Vβ chains.[31] IVIG may also downregulate expression of the accessory adhesion molecule lymphocyte function-associated antigen-1 (LFA-1) on activated T cells (*Fig. 1.10*).[32]

Intravenous immunoglobulin has also been reported to contain antibodies capable of neutralizing superantigens of bacterial and viral origin.[33] Such superantigens can broadly stimulate large numbers of beta-chain-expressing T cells that might trigger acute immunoinflammatory episodes in diseases such as MS, GBS or CIDP.

Restoration of a disturbed TH1/TH2 cytokine balance

T cells exert many of their actions through cytokines. These cytokines, based on their proinflammatory or antiinflammatory/down-regulatory actions can be classified into TH1 cytokines and TH2 cytokines. There is evidence to suggest that the inflammatory aspect of central nervous system demyelination in MS is associated with a preponderance of TH1 cytokines (IFNγ, IL-2, TNFα, lymphotoxin) released from a special subpopulation of CD4 T cells. Conversely, the remission phase of MS is characterized by enhanced generation of TH2 cytokines such as IL-4, IL-10 and TGFβ. IVIG may redress the disturbed balance by supplying neutralizing antibodies which bind TH1 cytokines, cytokine antagonists and contaminating TH2 cytokines such as TGFβ.[16,34-40] Experiments in vitro indicate that the addition of IVIG suppresses generation of TH1 cytokines and enhances production of TH1 cytokine antagonists and TH2 cytokines by T lymphocytes (*Fig. 1.10*).[41]

Inhibition of cell adhesion

Recently, IVIG has been reported to contain antibodies directed to the Arg-Gly-Asp (RGD) motif and the attachment site of a number of adhesive extracellular matrix proteins, including ligands for β1, β3 and β5 integrins.[42] It is therefore conceivable that IVIG may also affect the migration of immune cells from blood to brain.

Modulation of apoptosis

Intravenous immunoglobulin has been shown to inhibit the proliferation of activated T and B lymphocytes, and to induce programmed cell death in leukaemic cells of lymphocyte and monocyte lineage and in CD40-activated normal B cells.[43] This action involves, at least in part, Fas(CD95/Apo-1) pathways. It is theoretically conceivable that IVIG may promote cell death of autoreactive T lymphocytes. On the other hand, IVIG has also been shown to contain antibodies blocking Fas(CD95) mechanisms, which has been invoked in the therapeutic efficacy of IVIG in toxic epidermal necrolysis.

Possible effects on remyelination

In addition to terminating an acute inflammatory process or modulating aberrant immune responses, IVIG has also been invoked to promote remyelination in animal models of multiple sclerosis and GBS, experimental allergic encephalomyelitis (EAE) and experimental autoimmune neuritis (EAN).[44-48] However, it should be noted that in Theiler's virus-induced EAE in SJL mice,

IgM antibodies were much more potent than IgG in stimulating remyelination.

Conclusion

Intravenous immunoglobulin has been proved to be efficacious in the treatment of a number of immune-mediated neuromuscular disorders and possibly multiple sclerosis. In all likelihood, IVIG is a super-cocktail of immunoglobulins of various specificities and of contaminating immunologically active molecules that act at multiple sites in the disturbed immune system of patients afflicted with these disorders (see *Fig. 1.10*). In all likelihood, though, only some of the many potential actions may be clinically relevant.

References

1. Dalakas MC. The use of intravenous immunoglobulin for neurologic diseases. *Neurology* 1998; **51**(suppl 5).

2. Stangel M, Hartung HP, Marx P, Gold R. Intravenous immunoglobulin treatment of neurological autoimmune diseases. *J Neurol Sci* 1998; **153**:203–214.

3. Stangel M, Toyka KV, Gold R. Mechanisms of high-dose intravenous immunoglobulins in demyelinating diseases. *Arch Neurol* 1999; **56**: 661–663.

4. Roux KH, Tankersley DL. A view of the human idiotypic repertoire: electron microscopic and immunologic analyses of spontaneous idiotype-antiidiotype dimers in pooled human IgG. *J Immunol* 1990; **144**: 1387–1395.

5. Diegel M, Rankin B, Bolen J, Dubois P, Kiener P. Cross linking of Fc receptor to surface immunoglobulin on B cells provides an inhibitory signal that closes the plasma membrane calcium channel. *J Biol Chem* 1994; **269**: 11409–11416.

6. Jungi TW, Nydegger VE. Proposed mechanisms of action of intravenous IgG in autoimmune diseases. *Transfus Sci* 1992; **13**: 267–290.

7. Kondo N, Kasahara K, Kameyama T et al. Intravenous immunoglobulins suppress immunoglobulin production by suppressing $Ca(2+)$-dependent signal transduction through Fcγ receptors in B lymphocytes. *Scand J Immunol* 1994; **40**: 37–42.

8. Vassilev T, Gelin C, Kaveri SV et al. Antibodies to the CD5 molecule in normal human immunoglobulin for therapeutic use (intravenous immunoglobulins, IVIg). *Clin Exp Immunol* 1993; **92**: 369–372.

9. Kazatchkine MD, Dietrich G, Hurez V et al. V region-mediated selection of autoreactive repertoires by intravenous immunoglobulin. *Immunol Rev* 1994; **139**: 79–107.

10. Lacroix-Desmezes S, Kaveri SV, Mouthon L et al. Self-reactive antibodies (natural autoantibodies) in healthy individuals. *J Immunol Methods* 1998; **216**: 117–137.

11. Varela F, Andersson A, Dietrich G et al. The population dynamics of antibodies in normal and autoimmune individuals. *Proc Natl Acad Sci USA* 1991; **88**: 5917–5921.

12. Yu Z, Lennon VA. Mechanism of intravenous immune globulin therapy in antibody-mediated autoimmune diseases. *New Engl J Med* 1999; **340**: 227–228.

13. Yuki N, Miyaga F. Possible mechanism of intravenous immunoglobulin treatment on anti-GM1 antibody-mediated neuropathies. *J Neurol Sci* 1996; **139**: 160–162.

14. Dietrich G, Kazatchkine MD. Normal immunoglobulin G (IgG) for therapeutic use (intravenous Ig) contains anti-idiotypic specificities against an immunodominant, disease-associated, cross-reactive idiotype of human antithyroglobulin autoantibodies. *J Clin Invest* 1990; **85:** 620–629.

15. Hurez V, Kazatchkine MD, Vassilev T et al. Pooled normal human polyspecific IgG contains neutralizing anti-idiotypes to IgG autoantibodies of autoimmune patients and protects from experimental autoimmune disease. *Blood* 1997; **90:** 4004–4013.

16. Kaveri S, Prasad N, Vassilev T et al. Modulation of autoimmune responses by intravenous immunoglobulin. *Mult Scler* 1997; **3:** 121–128.

17. Tankersley DL, Preston MS, Finlayson JS. Immunoglobulin G dimer: an idiotype-antiidiotype complex. *Mol Immunol* 1988; **25:** 41–48.

18. Hartung HP, Pollard JD, Harvey GK, Toyka KV. Immunopathogenesis and treatment of the Guillain–Barré syndrome, Part II. *Muscle Nerve* 1995; **18:** 154–164.

19. Liblau R, Gajdos PH, Bustardet FA et al. Intravenous gamma globulin in myasthenia gravis: interaction with anti-acetylcholine receptor autoantibodies. *J Clin Immunol* 1991; **11:** 128–131.

20. Van Doorn PA, Brand A, Vermeulen M. Anti-neuroblastoma cell line antibodies in inflammatory demyelinating polyneuropathy: inhibition in vitro and in vivo by IV immunoglobulin. *Neurology* 1988; **38:** 1592–1595.

21. Lutz HU, Stammler P, Jelezarova E, Nater M, Späth PJ. High doses of immunoglobulin G attenuate immune aggregate-mediated complement activation by enhancing physiologic cleavage of C3b in C3bn-IgG complexes. *Blood* 1996; **88:** 184–193.

22. Basta M, Dalakas MC. High-dose intravenous immunoglobulin exerts its beneficial effect in patients with dermatomyositis by blocking endomysial deposition of activated complement fragments. *J Clin Invest* 1994; **94:** 1729–1735.

23. Basta M, Illa I, Dalakas MC. Increased in vitro uptake of the complement C3b in the serum of patients with Guillain Barré syndrome, myasthenia gravis and dermatomyositis. *J Neuroimmunol* 1996; **71:** 227–229.

24. Basta M, Kirshbom P, Frank MM, Fries LF. Mechanisms of therapeutic effect of high-dose intravenous immunoglobulin. *J Clin Invest* 1989; 1974–1981.

25. Dalakas MC. Mechanism of action of intravenous immunoglobulin and therapeutic considerations in the treatment of autoimmune neurologic diseases. *Neurology* 1998; **51(suppl):** S2–S8.

26. Fujii M, Koffmann B, Sivakumar K, Dalakas MC. Histopathologic characteristics in repeated muscle biopsies of patients with inclusion body myositis (IBM) treated in a control trial with high-dose intravenous immunoglobulin (IVIg) and prednisolone. *Neurology* 1997; **48:** 332–333.

27. Hartung HP, Toyka KV, Griffin JW. Guillain–Barré syndrome and chronic inflammatory demyelinating polyradiculoneuropathy. In: Antel J, Birnbaum G, Hartung HP, eds. *Clinical Neuroimmunology*. Malden: Blackwell Science, 1998, 294–306.

28, Malik U, Oleksowicz L, Latow N, Cardo LJ. Intravenous gamma-globulin inhibits binding of anti-GM1 to its target antigen. *Ann Neurol* 1996; **39:** 136–139.

29. Blasczyk R, Westhoff V, Grosse-Wilde H. Soluble CD4, CD8 and HLA molecules in commercial immunoglobulin preparations. *Lancet* 1993; **341**: 789–790.

30. Kaveri S, Vassilev T, Hurez V et al. Antibodies to a conserved region of HLA class I molecules, capable of modulating CD8 T cell-mediated function, are present in pooled normal immunoglobulin for therapeutic use. *J Clin Invest* 1996; **97**: 865–869.

31. Marchalonis JJ, Kaymaz H, Dedeoglu F et al. Human autoantibodies reactive with synthetic autoantigens from T cell receptor V beta chain. *Proc Natl Acad Sci USA* 1992; **89**: 3325–3329.

32. Rigal D, Vermot-Desroches C, Heitz S et al. Effect of IVIg in peripheral blood B, NK, and T cell subpopulations in women with recurrent spontaneous abortions: specific effect on LFA-1 and CD56 molecules. *Clin Immunol Immunopathol* 1994; **71**: 309–314.

33. Takei S, Arora YK, Walker SM. Intravenous immunoglobulin contains specific antibodies inhibitory of activation of T cells by staphylococcal toxin superantigens. *J Clin Invest* 1993; **91**: 602–607.

34. Abe Y, Horiuchi A, Miyake M, Kimura S. Anti-cytokine nature of natural human immunoglobulin: one possible mechanism of the clinical effect of intravenous immunoglobulin therapy. *Immunol Rev* 1994; **139**: 5–19.

35. Ankrust P, Muller F, Svenson M et al. Administration of intravenous immunoglobulin (IVIg) in vivo: downregulatory effects on the IL-1 system. *Clin Exp Immunol* 1999; **115**: 136–143.

36. Kekow J, Reinhold D, Pap T, Ansorge S. Intravenous immunoglobulins and transforming growth factor beta. *Lancet* 1998; **351**: 184–185.

37. Mansmann PT, Ong SH. Interferon content of intravenous immunoglobulin: variation between preparations. *Ped Asthma Allergy Immunol* 1997; **11**: 137–139.

38. Pashov A, Dubey C, Kaveri SV et al. Normal immunoglobulin G protects against experimental allergic encephalomyelitis by inducing transferable T cell unresponsiveness to myelin basic protein. *Eur J Immunol* 1998; **28**: 1823–1831.

39. Stangel M, Schumacher HC, Ruprecht K et al. Immunoglobulins for intravenous use inhibit TNFα cytotoxicity in vitro. *Immunol Invest* 1997; **26**: 569–578.

40. Svenson M, Hansen MB, Bendtzen K. Binding of cytokines to pharmaceutically prepared human immunoglobulin. *J Clin Invest* 1993; **92**: 2533–2539.

41. Pashov A, Bellon B, Kaveri SV, Kazatchkine MD. A shift in encephalitogenic T cell cytokine pattern is associated with suppression of EAE by intravenous immunoglobulins (IVIg). *Mult Scler* 1997; **3**: 153–156.

42. Vassilev TL, Kazatchkine MD, van Huyen JP et al. Inhibition of cell adhesion by antibodies to Arg-Gly-Asp (RGD) in normal immunoglobulin for therapeutic use (intravenous immunoglobulin, IVIg). *Blood* 1999; **93**: 3624–3631.

43. Prasad NK, Papoff G, Zeuner A et al. Therapeutic preparations of normal polyspecific IgG (IVIg) induce apoptosis in human lymphocytes and monocytes: a novel mechanism of action of IVIg involving the Fas apoptotic pathways. *J Immunol* 1998; **161**: 3781–3790.

44. Asakura K, Miller DJ, Murray K et al. Monoclonal autoantibody SCH94.03, which promotes central nervous system remyelination, recognizes an antigen on the

surface of oligodendrocytes. *J Neurosci Res* 1996; **43**: 273–281.

45. Enders U, Toyka KV, Hartung HP, Gold R. Failure of intravenous immunoglobulin (IVIg) therapy in experimental autoimmune neuritis (EAN) of the Lewis rat. *J Neuroimmunol* 1997; **76**: 112–116.

46. Gabriel CM, Gregson NA, Redford EJ et al. Human immunoglobulin ameliorates rat experimental allergic neuritis. *Brain* 1997; **120**: 1533–1540.

47. Rodriguez M. Central nervous system demyelination and remyelination in multiple sclerosis and viral models of disease. *J Neuroimmunol* 1992; **40**: 255–264.

48. Van Engelen BGM, Miller DJ, Pavelko KD et al. Promotion of remyelination by polyclonal immunoglobulin in Theiler's virus-induced demyelination and in multiple sclerosis. *J Neurol Neurosurg Psychiatry* 1994; **57**(**suppl**): 65–68.

Multifocal neuropathies

2

Richard A Lewis

> ALS: amyotrophic lateral sclerosis; CIDP: chronic inflammatory demyelinating polyradiculoneuropathy; CNS: central nervous system; CSF: cerebrospinal fluid; DLR: diabetic lumbosacral radiculoplexoneuropathy; ELISA: enzyme-linked immunosorbent assay; HIV: human immunodeficiency virus; Ig: immunoglobulin; IVIG: intravenous immunoglobulin; LSS: Lewis–Sumner syndrome; LMND: lower motor neuron disorder; MAG: myelin associated glycoprotein; MMN: multifocal motor neuropathy; MSMDN, multifocal sensorimotor demyelinating neuropathy: POEMS: polyneuropathy, orgonomegaly, endocrinopathy, m-protein skin disorder; UMN: upper motor neuron

Introduction

Intravenous immunoglobulin (IVIG) has become an important therapeutic option in the treatment of inflammatory and autoimmune neuropathies. Many of these present as a symmetric disorder despite the fact that they are caused by multifocal attacks on the peripheral nervous system. However, there are certain disorders in which the clinical history and examination reveal a pattern of multiple involvement of individual nerves, or are so strikingly asymmetric, that the multifocal character helps define the disorder. The term *mononeuropathy* (or *mononeuritis*) *multiplex* is used to describe neuropathies that evolve by damaging individual nerves in a random fashion such that on careful examination the individual nerves involved can be readily identified. The term *confluent mononeuropathy multiplex* is used when so many nerves have become involved that it may not be possible to identify the specific nerve insults on examination, although frequently a careful history will point to the evolution of the individual nerve attacks.

Prior to 1980, the known causes of mononeuritis multiplex were primarily confined to the collagen vascular disorders and vasculitides. However, since then a number of other disorders have been recognized (*Table 2.1*). Vasculitis is known to cause an ischemic insult of peripheral nerve with wallerian degeneration as the pathologic consequence of the nerve infarct. Along with collagen vascular and vasculitic disorders, diabetes mellitus has been frequently mentioned as a cause of mononeuritis multiplex, but there are few, if any, descriptions of a diabetic mononeuropathy multiplex that involves the upper extremities unrelated to compression palsies. Specific focal and multifocal disorders related to diabetes, such as diabetic amyotrophy, truncal radiculopathy and cranial mononeuropathies, have been considered to be caused by ischemic insults due to microvascular occlusive disease. Recent evidence is pointing to an inflammatory, possibly vasculitic disorder, as the cause of the multifocal diabetic neuropathies. The potential for antiinflammatory and immunomodulating treatments to influence the course of these disorders is now being reconsidered.

In 1982, five patients were described who had a sensorimotor mononeuropathy multiplex, but rather than prominent wallerian degeneration, the expected finding in vasculitic mononeuritis multiplex, these patients had striking and persistent multifocal conduction block and segmental demyelination.[1] The two patients who were treated with prednisone responded in a time frame consistent with recovery from conduction block rather than the slower time course of recovery from wallerian degeneration. These patients were described as having multifocal sensorimotor demyelinating neuropathy with persistent conduction block (MSMDN) and were considered to have a variant of chronic inflammatory demyelinating polyradiculoneuropathy (CIDP) which had previously been described as a symmetric disorder.

In 1988 Parry and Clarke[2]—and in a

Table 2.1
Causes of mononeuropathy multiplex.

Demyelinating neuropathies
Multifocal motor neuropathy with persistent conduction block
Multifocal sensorimotor demyelinating neuropathy with persistent conduction block (Lewis–Sumner syndrome)
Hereditary neuropathy with predisposition to pressure palsies

Vasculitic and ischemic neuropathies
Systemic lupus erythematosus
Rheumatoid vasculitis
Systemic sclerosis (scleroderma)
Periarteritis nodosa
Churg–Strauss syndrome
Wegener's granulomatosis
Paraneoplastic vasculitic neuropathy
Nonsystemic vasculitic neuropathy
Behçet syndrome
Giant cell arteritis

Diabetes mellitus
Lumbosacral radiculoplexopathy
Truncal radiculopathy
Cranial mononeuropathies
Sensory perineuritis

Infectious neuropathies
Leprosy
Herpes zoster
Lyme disease
HIV-associated cytomegalovirus
Hepatitis C and cryoglobulinemia

Other causes
Sarcoid
Brachial neuritis (Parsonage–Turner syndrome)
Monomelic amyotrophy
Malignant infiltration of peripheral nerve
Neurofibromatosis

separate report, Pestronk et al[3]—reported patients who were initially considered to have lower motor neuron forms of amyotrophic lateral sclerosis (ALS), but were found to have a motor mononeuropathy multiplex related to persistent conduction block. Since then, there have been a number of studies describing patients with multifocal motor neuropathy with persistent conduction block (MMN). Whether patients with MMN and patients with MSMDN have the same disorder with varying degrees of sensory involvement has been debated and the term Lewis–Sumner syndrome has been used interchangeably by different authors to describe both entities. Recent reports have suggested significant differences between these two disorders which may have important therapeutic and pathophysiologic significance. For this reason, the two disorders are considered separately in this chapter and the term Lewis–Sumner syndrome (LSS) is used to describe only the sensorimotor disorder.

Intravenous immunoglobulin has been considered as a potential therapeutic option for many of the multifocal disorders. The treatment of mononeuritis multiplex due to vasculitis and other systemic disorders is based on treating the underlying medical condition. The role of IVIG in these disorders remains unclear and is outside the scope of this chapter. This discussion is confined to a review of MMN, MSMDN (LSS) and diabetic mononeuropathies.

Multifocal motor neuropathy with persistent conduction block

Background

Most reviews point to the reports in 1988 of Parry and Clarke[2] and of Pestronk et al[3] as identifying MMN. However, there were earlier reports in which the various aspects of the disorder were described.[4-7] The two 1988 reports described patients who were initially considered to have lower motor neuron forms of ALS but were found to have a multifocal demyelinating neuropathy. Parry's five cases and Pestronk's two cases all presented with multifocal weakness, atrophy, cramps and fasciculations without significant sensory complaints. Parry and Clarke emphasized that the symptoms began in the arms, that reflexes were usually normal or lost focally, that cerebrospinal fluid (CSF) protein was normal and the course was slowly progressive. Treatment responses were variable. One patient did not respond to plasmapheresis, one stabilized when azathioprine was added to prednisone and one patient did not respond to plasmapheresis, prednisone or cyclophosphamide. The cardinal feature of the disorder was multifocal conduction block and conduction slowing which appeared to be confined to motor nerve fibers. Distal sensory responses were normal and somatosensory evoked responses and compound nerve action potentials were normal across the regions of motor block.

Pestronk also emphasized the early involvement of the upper limbs, the presence of fasciculations, the lack of upper motor neuron signs or bulbar involvement and the normal sensory examination. The level of CSF protein was elevated to 69 mg/dl (0.69 g/l) in one patient and was normal in the other. There were similar findings of motor conduction block as well as conduction slowing with normal distal sensory conduction. Sural nerve biopsy was normal in one patient and revealed occasional wallerian-like degeneration in another. A motor point biopsy showed axonal loss and demyelination of the remaining axons. There was no significant response to treatment with prednisone or plasmapheresis but both patients responded to intravenous and/or oral cyclophosphamide. Both patients had IgM antibodies that reacted with GM1 ganglioside. The titers of the anti-GM1 antibodies fell after cyclophosphamide treatment.

Both reports mention that some of the patients had mild and vague sensory symptoms but no significant abnormality on clinical examination and sensory conduction studies were normal. Since these reports, there have been a number of case reports and small series that have defined the clinical syndrome and the electrophysiologic features. They have addressed the controversial issue of the significance of elevated titers of anti-GM1 antibody and response to various treatments. In particular, many authors have emphasized intravenous immunoglobulin in the treatment of MMN.

Clinical features

Multifocal motor neuropathy is a rare motor disorder that is more common in men than women. While it is difficult to determine an accurate figure from the multiple reports, combining the data from some of the larger series suggests a male to female ratio of at least 2 : 1.[8-11] The age range has been reported as 20–70 years, with most patients aged 25–55 years. The disease usually progresses slowly, with some reports mentioning disease progression of over 20 years.[8,10] However, some patients will have a more aggressive decline.[3,7,9]

Patients frequently are misdiagnosed as having a lower motor neuron form of amyotrophic lateral sclerosis. Painless, asymmetric weakness, atrophy and fasciculations of the upper extremities are usually the presenting features. On occasion, the symptoms can be isolated to one or two nerves. Despite marked lower motor neuron changes, sensory symptoms never are prominent, although some patients describe vague sensory phenomena or intermittent mild sensory symptoms. Discrete sensory symptoms in the distribution of the motor complaints are not present. Atrophy, fasciculations, myokymia and cramps are seen in various combinations.[7,10] Tinel's signs at the sites of the conduction block have not been mentioned. While the legs may become involved, they rarely are the first limb involved and the severity of the disease is usually less in the legs, so that the patient may remain ambulatory despite severe upper extremity weakness. Focal hemiatrophy of the tongue has been described[12] but bulbar and pseudobulbar dysfunction have not been reported. Sensory examination is almost always normal, even in patients with sensory symptoms. However, some reports mention distal vibration sense reduction[3] or sensory symptoms later in the course.[2] Deep tendon reflexes tend to be preserved out of proportion to the weakness. They can be lost focally, particularly in the arms, but it is unusual to have complete areflexia unless the weakness has become generalized and profound. Some reports mention relative hyperreflexia[3] but Babinski responses or sustained clonus pointing to upper motor neuron (UMN) involvement are not seen. Lange et al[13] addressed the issue of whether UMN signs can clinically distinguish ALS from MMN. They found motor conduction block (10 patients) or focal temporal dispersion (seven patients) in 17 patients out of 169 patients with motor neuron disease. One patient out of the 10 patients with conduction block had Babinski signs or sustained clonus, while five others had incongruously brisk reflexes. Three of the seven patients with no block but temporal dispersion had definite upper motor neuron signs and two had brisk reflexes. The implications of this study are that conduction block, as opposed to temporal dispersion, appears to best define the syndrome of MMN and that true UMN signs are rare in patients with MMN, but brisk reflexes may be seen. The diagnosis of MMN should be questioned in patients with otherwise unexplained UMN signs.

Electrodiagnostic features

The defining feature of MMN is motor conduction block. Conduction block occurs when saltatory transmission is focally blocked. Most clinical disorders that are related to conduction block are due to structural or physiologic changes at nodes of Ranvier and are associated with segmental demyelination. Pathologic investigations of peripheral nerve in tourniquet-induced conduction block[14] and in intraneural injection of antigalactocerebroside serum[15,16] have demonstrated the pathophysiologic features of conduction block. While segmental demyelination does not need to be present for conduction block to be present, segmental demyelination will eventually occur,[16] and virtually all clinical conditions causing conduction block are associated with segmental demyelination. The underlying axon is normal in lesions causing conduction block. While secondary wallerian degeneration can occur, the demonstration of conduction block requires that the amplitude of the motor response on stimulation proximal to the lesion must be substantially less than on stimulation distal to the lesion (*Fig. 2.1*). The criteria for determining conduction block remains a source of controversy. Amplitude reductions ranging from 20% to 60% have been used in reports of MMN.[17,18] The amplitude reduction cannot be secondary to temporal dispersion, and in an attempt to demonstrate this many investigators will determine if the area under the negative peak also has a significant reduction. If the reduction in area under the negative peak on proximal stimulation compared with distal stimulation is less than the degree of reduction in amplitude, this would imply that at least some of the amplitude reduction is due to temporal

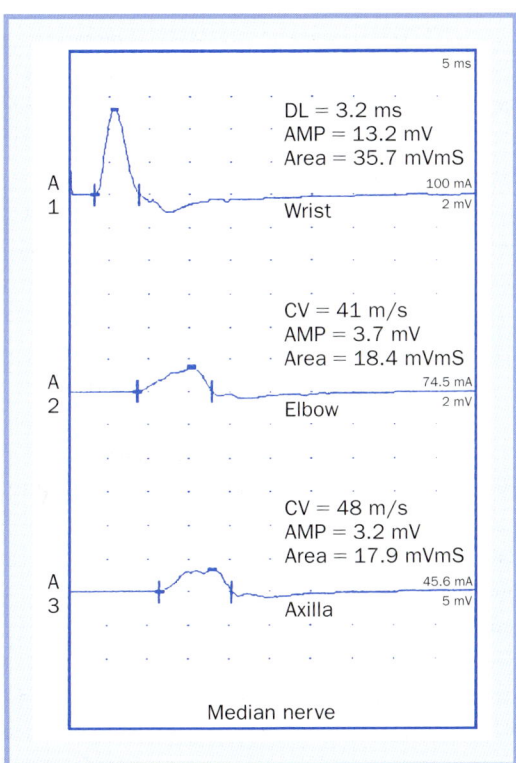

Figure 2.1
Motor conduction block without temporal dispersion.

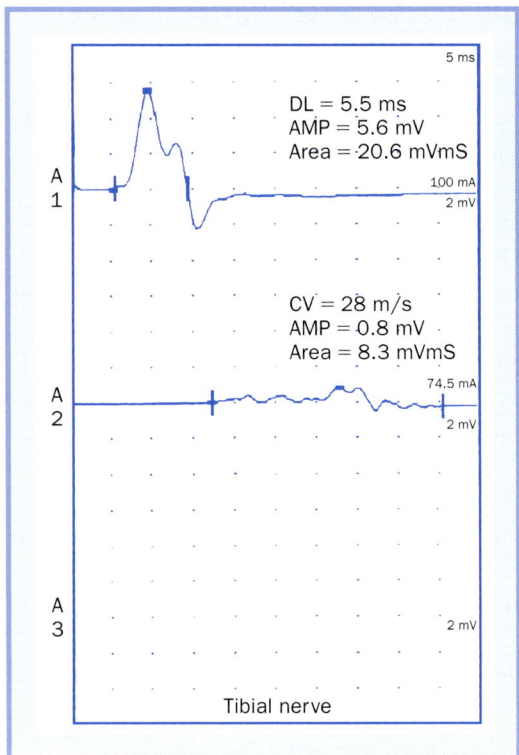

Figure 2.2
Temporal dispersion. The reduced area suggests partial conduction block along with the temporal dispersion.

dispersion (*Fig. 2.2*). In addition, temporal dispersion can produce phase cancellation further reducing the amplitude on proximal stimulation.[19] Therefore, while it is theoretically possible for amplitude reductions as small as 20% to be due to conduction block, in reality there are too many other causes of reduced amplitude to utilize this criteria. Most authors recommend criteria of approximately 50% reduction in both amplitude and area to determine conduction block with less than 20% increase in duration.[20]

While conduction block is the defining electrophysiologic feature of MMN, other electrodiagnostic features of segmental demyelination have been noted.[9,20–23] These include prolonged distal motor latencies, prolonged F wave latencies, multifocally slow motor conduction velocities and temporal dispersion. In most instances conduction block is detected in at least one nerve, along with the other features of demyelination. These findings may be in nerves without conduction block. Whether the diagnosis of MMN can be made without evidence of conduction block remains in question. The inability to detect conduction block may be due to difficulties stimulating above and below very proximal or very distal lesions or may be due to secondary wallerian degeneration masking the primary conduction block lesion. It is reasonable to strongly consider MMN in patients with an appropriate clinical picture and electrodiagnostic evidence of segmental demyelination but without conduction block. However, response to treatment does not appear to be as good in these patients as with those with conduction block.

Sensory conduction studies are normal in MMN. Those investigators that have attempted to look for sensory conduction changes in the regions of motor block have been unable to detect any abnormality utilizing sensory conduction, compound nerve action potentials and somatosensory evoked responses.[2,12,20,24]

Laboratory features

The CSF protein tends to be normal or only mildly elevated,[11] reflecting the minimal involvement of nerve roots. There are no other significant abnormalities on routine spinal fluid or serum testing.

The most significant, albeit controversial, laboratory finding in many patients with MMN is the presence of elevated titers of antibody against GM1 ganglioside. GM1 is one of a number of gangliosides that are constituents of cell membranes and have been implicated in neuroimmunologic disorders. GM1, GD1a, GD1b, GT1a and GT1b constitute over 80% of the total gangliosides in most mammalian brains[25] and GM1 is the most abundant ganglioside in human central nervous system (CNS) myelin.[26] The GM1 epitope is present in motor neurons and their axons and to a lesser extent in dorsal root ganglion cells and sensory axons,[27] but there may be differences in the ceramide composition of GM1 in motor and sensory axons.[28] While the amount of GM1 in peripheral nerve is minimal, it is a major peripheral nerve antigen, found at nodes of Ranvier and also on the axolemma.[29] The mechanism by which anti-GM1 antibodies might cause conduction block remains unclear. The possibility that the antibodies cause blockade of sodium channels[30,31] has been challenged[27] and an alternate explanation has been given. Hyperpolarization of nerve fiber membranes mediated by potassium channels has been suggested as a mechanism of increasing nodal threshold to the point of producing conduction block.

The incidence of anti-GM1 antibodies in MMN is not entirely clear. Some reports mention only 20% incidence while others report high titers in over 80%.[32] The reason for this discrepancy is probably multifactorial. It remains unclear what degree of elevation of titers should be considered significant. It is clear that the specificity increases if only very high titers are designated as significant. Different laboratories use different techniques, and not all laboratories use the same disease controls, making it difficult to compare the results from different laboratories. Pestronk and Choksi[32] reported that 85% of patients with MMN had elevated titers to GM1 combined with other lipids including galactocerebroside and cholesterol while no patient with ALS had elevated titers. This combination appeared to increase the sensitivity and maintain the specificity of the antibodies. However, Carpo et al, utilizing the same technique, noted elevated titers in only 35% of patients with MMN, although this was an increase from 31% found with the standard ELISA technique.[33] However, the specificity was slightly decreased. Thus the sensitivity of IgM anti-GM1 antibodies remains variable, possibly laboratory-dependent. The specificity has also been variable but most of the recent studies have found high titers primarily in MMN and rarely in ALS, CIDP or other neurologic disorders. In a metaanalysis, van Schaik et al[34] noted that different methodologies, particularly the use of detergent and the duration and temperature of incubation, significantly influenced results. The ELISA methods utilizing no detergent and longer incubation periods resulted in a specificity of 90% and sensitivity of 38% in the comparison of MMN with other lower motor neuron disorders. The probability of MMN if titers were highly raised was between 50% and 85%, considered to be clinically significant. While there is evidence that anti-GM1 antibodies have the potential for causing conduction block and demyelination,[35] there is still no clear evidence that the antibodies are the specific cause of MMN. Thus, the current state of knowledge points to a correlation between high-titer anti-GM1 antibodies and MMN which is rarely seen in ALS or other neurologic disorders. However, the specificity and sensitivity of high titers are probably not strong enough to make detection of high-titer antibodies diagnostic in and of themselves. At best, they may be confirmatory of the diagnosis of MMN when the clinical and/or electrophysiologic findings are unclear. High-titer antibodies in patients with other diagnoses may encourage the clinician to reevaluate the situation and reconsider MMN. On occasion, the detection of high-titer antibody may suggest an empiric trial of immunotherapy in a patient with otherwise untreatable conditions. It may be very difficult for a treating physician not to consider IVIG in a patient with possible or probable ALS but who also has high titers of anti-GM1 antibodies. Van den Berg et al[36] treated five patients with lower motor neuron disorders (LMND) who had high titers of anti-GM1 antibodies but who did not have conduction block. Only one of these patients responded to IVIG and the benefit did not persist with chronic treatment. The authors concluded that the presence of high titers of anti-GM1 antibodies did not identify a subgroup of patients with lower motor neuron syndromes, atypical of MMN, who would respond to IVIG. Similarly, Azulay et al[37] showed, in a placebo-controlled, crossover trial in 12 patients with LMND and high titers of anti-GM1 antibodies, that only the five patients with conduction block responded. Tsai et al[38] reported that 12 patients with LMND and elevated anti-GM1 antibody titers without conduction block did not clinically improve with intravenous cyclophosphamide despite reductions in antibody titers. Pestronk et al,[39] on the other hand, noted improvement in four patients with LMND and high-titer anti-GM1 antibodies without conduction block when treated with plasmapheresis and cyclophosphamide. While it is enticing to consider immunomodulating and/or immunosuppressant treatment in atypical cases of lower motor neuron disorders, experience suggests that one cannot be overly optimistic about success.

Treatment

Intravenous immunoglobulin has been shown to be effective in both controlled and uncontrolled trials and is considered as the initial treatment of choice.[37,40–42] Most patients will show improvement after the initial treatment at 2 g/kg in divided doses with functional benefit in over 50%.[8] However, less than 10% will maintain benefit for a year after one treatment and most patients require intermittent dosing to sustain functional recovery. As in the treatment of other chronic neuroimmunologic disorders, most patients require a modified dosage every 3–6 weeks. Some patients do best with a low dose weekly while others can be maintained with higher doses on a monthly basis. The treatment needs to be individualized and the dosing titrated slowly. The lowest possible dose at the longest interval that maximizes function is the goal of most clinicians. This approach minimizes the cost and inconvenience to the patient without compromising the clinical status of the patient.

The expectations of the physician and patient need to be realistic. A muscle with significant denervation on electromyography pointing to secondary wallerian degeneration is not going to improve quickly and is less likely to have complete recovery. It is also known that demyelinating conduction block lesions may take over 4 weeks to recover.[14,15]

Therefore, lack of improvement after an initial treatment does not necessarily mean treatment failure. Most clinicians would treat for 2–3 months before abandoning IVIG as therapy. However, if a patient develops a new conduction block lesion during treatment, then alternative therapies should be considered.

It may not be necessary to treat every patient with MMN. With greater recognition of this disorder, patients are being diagnosed earlier and some may have very few lesions and minimal functional deficit. In addition, the disorder may be very slow and intermittent with long periods of inactivity. In these instances, it may be prudent to withhold treatment until active conduction block lesions develop or functional disability occurs.

It is important to monitor treatment carefully. Quantitative muscle testing and functional assessments may be helpful. Repeat electrodiagnostic studies frequently show at least partial reversal of the conduction block. There has been some discrepancy between clinical improvement and electrophysiologic improvement, although it is difficult to understand how strength could improve without the conduction block improving.

Unfortunately, not all patients benefit from IVIG and new regions of conduction block or progressive axonal loss during treatment have been documented.[40,43] Alternative treatments that have documented benefit are relatively few. Both oral[11,44–46] and high-dose intravenous[47] corticosteroid treatment have been remarkably ineffective. The few reports of plasmapheresis treatment without other medications have also not been encouraging.[2]

Cyclophosphamide is the only immunosuppressive agent that has been reported to be effective.[39,46,48,49] Most of the published regimens utilize intravenous cyclophosphamide but there is no consensus on the optimal treatment program. Nobile-Orazio[49] used relatively low daily doses (1.5–3 mg/kg) of oral cyclophosphamide on two patients and felt that the frequency of IVIG treatments could be reduced. Pestronk,[48] in a review article without published data, recommended six monthly treatments at 1 g/m^2 preceded by two plasma exchanges. In his experience, this reduced the serum anti-GM1 titer in 60–80% of patients with functional benefit in some of these. Pestronk states that the remission can last for 1–3 years but relapse frequently occurs and retreatment may be necessary. The risks of cyclophosphamide are well known and include bone marrow suppression, risk of opportunistic infection and an increased risk of neoplasia. It is important to determine whether the possible benefits warrant taking the inherent risks of cyclophosphamide treatment.

Multifocal sensorimotor demyelinating neuropathy: Lewis–Sumner syndrome

In 1982, Lewis, Sumner, Brown and Asbury[1] reported five patients who had a sensorimotor mononeuropathy multiplex. All five had symptoms that included pain and numbness as well as weakness in multiple nerve distributions. Motor neuron disease would not have been considered in the differential diagnosis of any of these patients. Two patients had episodes of optic neuritis with central scotomas, afferent pupillary defects, and prolonged visual evoked responses. Cerebrospinal fluid protein was normal or mildly increased. Sural nerve biopsy revealed segmental demyelination and a small amount of inflammatory cell infiltrate. Two patients treated with corticosteroids improved. The unique finding in these patients, which distinguished them from patients with vasculitic mononeuritis multiplex, was the presence of conduction block, which in some cases was demonstrated to persist for many years.

Prior to 1995, the disorder was mostly either ignored or lumped with MMN. However, since then there have been a few series of patients with sensorimotor symptoms.[11,50] These reports, consistent with the original LSS patients, suggest differences between the patients with pure motor symptoms and those with sensory and motor symptoms. The increased incidence of MMN in males is not noted in MSMDN. Pain, paresthesias and Tinel's signs are only seen in patients with sensory symptoms. Sural nerve biopsies of patients with MSMDN reveal significantly more abnormalities consistent with a demyelinating neuropathy than do biopsies of patients with MMN.[11,50,51] High titers of GM1 antibodies have not been reported in MSMDN, although Oh noted one patient out of 16 with mildly elevated titers. Cerebrospinal fluid protein, while not very elevated, tends to be higher than in patients with MMN, suggesting that nerve roots may be more involved in MSMDN. A significant number of patients with MSMDN respond to corticosteroids; 50% (3 of 6) in Saperstein's series and 79% (11 of 14) in Oh's series. This is in distinct contrast to patients with MMN, in whom corticosteroids have been remarkably ineffective. Most cases of MMN that were reported to respond to corticosteroids, at closer view, had sensory signs or symptoms and more probably were MSMDN.[52,53]

The findings on motor conduction studies in MSMDN are indistinguishable from those found in MMN. However, sensory abnormalities are usually seen, particularly if proximal stimulation is utilized. Whether the distal sensory response is abnormal depends on whether the conduction block lesion is distal, or whether secondary wallerian degeneration has occurred. However, most patients tend to show some distal sensory amplitude reduction.

In contradistinction to MMN, in which multiple reports have shown normal sensory conduction through areas of motor block, there is now at least one case of MSMDN demonstrating sensory conduction block which improved with treatment (*Fig. 2.3*).[54]

There does appear to be a 'gray zone' in which occasional patients cannot easily be labeled as having MMN or MSMDN. Parry notes that he has seen patients who present with a pure motor syndrome but then develop sensory symptoms years later. It is also apparent that some patients have a few sensory symptoms or minor changes on sensory conduction studies and it becomes difficult to decide whether these changes are significant enough to warrant a diagnosis of MSMDN. These are reasons why some investigators suggest 'lumping' MMN and MSMDN together as a single entity. Although it will be necessary to identify more patients with both MMN and MSMDN before one can determine if the distinctions mentioned above are significant, it appears prudent to separate the two disorders. First of all, the lumping together of the two disorders potentially confuses the issue of GM1 antibodies. The true incidence of these antibodies in MMN will never be known if patients with MSMDN are included. Most importantly, there appears to be a real difference in response to corticosteroid therapy. The potential benefits of long-term prednisone in MSMDN may outweigh the risks. However, there is currently no evidence to support the use of corticosteroids in MMN.

Intravenous immunoglobulin has also been shown to be of benefit in some patients with MSMDN. Saperstein noted a 56% response to IVIG (five of nine patients). Two patients did not respond to IVIG or prednisone. Oh noted 50% of patients did not respond to IVIG (three of six). The regimen is not likely to differ from that utilized for MMN. Whether patients respond better to IVIG than to corticosteroids is not yet clear. The response to plasmapheresis is not known nor are there enough reports to determine if cyclosporin, azathioprine or cyclophosphamide have any role in the treatment of this relatively rare disorder.

Most authors have suggested that MSMDN is a form of CIDP[1,11,50] and some investigators wonder whether the disorder should be considered separately from CIDP. One could make a similar argument about MMN. It is increasingly clear that CIDP is not a single disorder, but like its cousin, Guillain–Barré syndrome, CIDP should also be considered a syndrome with many subgroups including MMN, MSMDN, POEMS, anti-MAG neuropathy, the neuropathies associated with monoclonal gammopathies, and sensory predominant CIDP. Recognition of these different disorders will hopefully provide clues that will unravel the immunopathologic causes of these disorders.

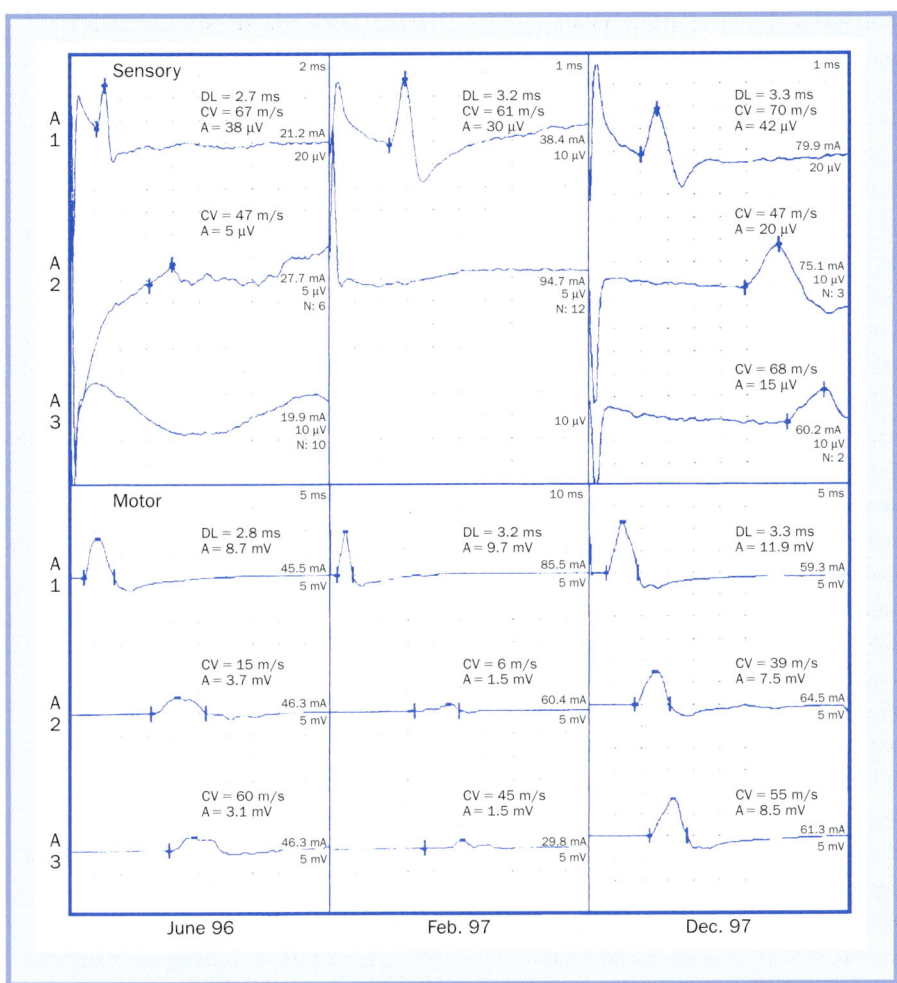

Figure 2.3
Motor and sensory conduction block with improvement after therapy given between February and December 1997.

Diabetic radiculoplexopathies and multifocal neuropathies

Diabetic distal symmetric sensory predominant neuropathy is the most common neuropathy in the world. This is a slowly progressive disorder with an incidence that increases with the duration of the diabetes. It is also known that diabetic patients are predisposed to mononeuropathies at typical sites of compression, such as the ulnar nerve at the elbow and the median nerve at the wrist.

In addition, diabetic patients also are predisposed to other focal and multifocal disorders. These include cranial mononeuropathies, thoracic radiculopathies, and lumbosacral radiculoplexopathies. Their cause is not yet known, but recent information has caused a reevaluation of the origins and treatment of these disorders. Most of the reports have been about lumbosacral radiculoplexopathy, but it is likely that the information gathered about this disorder has important implications regarding thoracic radiculopathies and some of the cranial mononeuropathies. There are many features in common in these disorders. They all present with pain, are usually subacute in progression and at least partially resolve over a period of 3–12 months. They tend to occur mostly in type II diabetes and both the thoracic and lumbosacral disorders may have weight loss as part of the syndrome.

The most frequent cranial nerve palsies seen in people with diabetes are the oculomotor, abducens and facial nerve palsies, although whether the incidence of some of these is significantly greater in diabetic than in nondiabetic subjects has been debated. Diabetic oculomotor neuropathy has been the most carefully studied.[55,56] Clinically, patients present with periorbital pain and then quickly develop weakness in muscles innervated by cranial nerve III including levator palpebrae, but pupillary constriction is not involved. This pupillary sparing helps to distinguish diabetic nerve III palsy from lesions caused by aneurysms or other space-occupying lesions. Typically patients spontaneously recover most function over 3–6 months. In a carefully done autopsy study, Asbury et al[55] showed significant microvascular disease primarily involving intraneural vessels with hyaline thickening and luminal narrowing. One extraneural vessel was occluded. Of interest was that the pathologic process appeared to be demyelinating, which was felt to be on an ischemic basis. No inflammatory infiltrates were detected.

Pain in the abdomen or chest, frequently described as burning, stabbing or aching, is the chief complaint of patients with diabetic thoracic radiculopathy. Radicular radiation is not typical but can be an important clue to diagnosis when it is present. The symptoms frequently mimic those of thoracic zoster but without the vesicular skin lesions. Patients may have significant weight loss, which frequently leads to an evaluation for possible malignancy. Electromyographic findings of denervation in thoracic paraspinal muscles point to the neuropathic disorder. Recovery usually occurs spontaneously but may take as long as 2 years.[57]

Diabetic lumbosacral radiculoplexoneuropathy (DLR) also first manifests as pain, most frequently in the hip and thigh. Weight loss, sometimes of a profound nature, may accompany the weakness and dysesthesias which usually begin in one limb but can become bilateral. Proximal muscles are most frequently involved, particularly in the femoral and obturator-innervated muscles. The disorder tends to progress over weeks but some progression has been reported over 6 months. Partial recovery over 12 months is anticipated in the majority of cases. The disorder was first described by Bruns over a hundred years ago and was entitled 'diabetic amyotrophy' by Garland.[58] It has also been called 'diabetic femoral neuropathy' and 'diabetic proximal neuropathy'. There has been confusion in the literature with patients who have a more chronic and symmetric disorder and have also been described as having diabetic amyotrophy.[59,60] The term DLR is therefore used here to describe the asymmetric disorder. A similar disorder has been shown to occur in nondiabetic patients[61,62] with virtually identical clinical features.

The cause of DLR remains unclear. The pathologic study of Raff and Asbury[63] demonstrated microvascular occlusive disease without inflammation very similar to the changes found in the oculomotor nerve. It was felt that this disorder, similar to the nerve III palsy, was due to diabetic microvascular occlusive disease as opposed to a metabolic derangement which was considered the likely cause of diabetic distal symmetric neuropathy. However, newer studies are raising questions about the etiologies of all the diabetic neuropathic disorders.

In particular, the possibility that DLR may be an inflammatory and/or immunologic disorder has been raised by a number of investigators. In 1984, Bradley et al[59] reported six patients with lumbosacral plexopathy with elevated erythrocyte sedimentation rate and epineural vasculitis who responded to immunosuppressive treatment. Three of these patients had diabetes. Said[64] biopsied the intermediate cutaneous nerve of the thigh in 10 patients with DLR and found vasculitis in two, inflammatory infiltrates in four and some evidence of segmental demyelination, along with axonal degeneration in most of the biopsies (Fig 2.4). Subsequent reports of diabetic and nondiabetic patients have shown similar results,[62,65,66] strongly implying an inflammatory microvascular vasculitis as a significant component of this disorder. Reports of sensory perineuritis in diabetic and nondiabetic patients as well as the possible predisposition of people with diabetes to

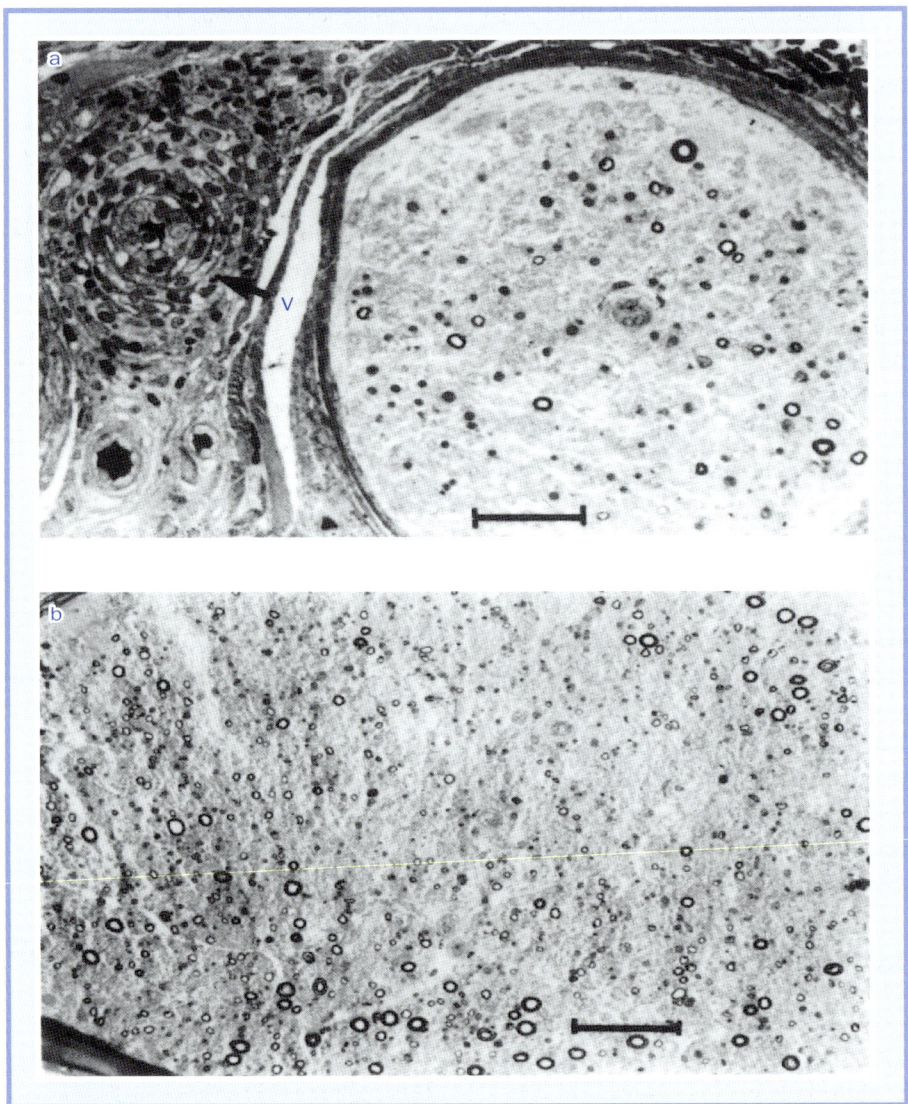

Figure 2.4
(a) Biopsy of intermediate cutaneous nerve of the thigh showing an inflammatory infiltrate around the perineural blood vessel and a reduction in nerve fibre density in the neighbouring fascicle. (b) Another fascicle showing axon loss indicative of recent ischaemia. Photographs supplied by Professor G Said and reproduced with permission from Lippincott–Williams and Wilkins.

CIDP all add credence to the possibility of an increased incidence of autoimmune and inflammatory neuropathies in diabetes.[67–71]

Studies of the efficacy of immunosuppressive and immunomodulating treatments in general, and IVIG in particular, in DLR are just beginning to emerge. Corticosteroids, plasmapheresis and IVIG have been reported, in small, uncontrolled series, to be of benefit,[65,73–76] but it is difficult to come to any conclusions at this time. Krendel treated 21 patients with immunosuppressors or immunomodulators including 16 patients who had IVIG as part of their regimen. Interestingly, while 11 of the patients had a lower extremity disorder consistent with DLR, four patients had thoracic radiculopathy and four had some asymmetric upper extremity involvement. Some of the reports suggest that there is a dramatic response in the resolution of pain in addition to what appears to be a more rapid recovery in motor function and improvement in disability. A placebo-controlled trial will hopefully determine whether the use of IVIG is beneficial in the majority of cases of DLR.

Conclusion

It is apparent that IVIG has an important role to play in the treatment of immune-mediated peripheral neuropathies. The disorders that present in a multifocal fashion are of particular interest in that they frequently can be misdiagnosed. Multifocal motor neuropathy often masquerades as a lower motor neuron form of ALS. Multifocal sensorimotor demyelinating neuropathy can mimic vasculitic mononeuritis multiplex and patients with diabetic thoracic and lumbosacral radiculoplexopathies (particularly when weight loss is present) often are initially considered to have malignancies. It is therefore crucial for the clinician to recognize these disorders so that the appropriate treatment can be given.

References

1. Lewis RA, Sumner AJ, Brown MJ, Asbury AK. Multifocal demyelinating neuropathy with persistent conduction block. *Neurology* 1982; **32:** 958–962.

2. Parry GJ, Clarke S. Multifocal acquired demyelinating neuropathy masquerading as motor neuron disease. *Muscle Nerve* 1988; **11:** 103–107.

3. Pestronk A, Cornblath DR, Ilyas AA et al. A treatable multifocal neuropathy with antibodies to GM1 ganglioside. *Ann Neurol* 1988; **24:** 73–78.

4. Chad DA, Hammer K, Sargent J. Slow resolution of multifocal weakness and fasciculation: a reversible motor neuron syndrome. *Neurology* 1982; **32:** 958–964.

5. Engel WK, Hopkins LC, Rosenberg BJ. Fasciculating progressive muscular atrophy (F-PMA) remarkably responsive to antidysimmune treatment (ADIT)—a possible clue to more ordinary ALS? *Neurology* 1985; **335 (suppl 1b):** 72.

6. Freddo L, Yu RK, Latov N et al. Gangliosides GM1 and GD1b are antigens for IgM M-protein in a patient with motor neuron disease. *Neurology* 1986; **36**: 454–458.

7. Roth G, Rohr J, Magistris MR, Oschner F. Motor neuropathy with proximal multifocal persistent block, fasciculations and myokymia. Evolution to tetraplegia. *Eur Neurol* 1986; **25**: 416–423.

8. Bouche P, Moulonguet A, Ben Younes-Chennnoufi A et al. Multifocal motor neuropathy with conduction block: a study of 24 patients. *J Neurol Neurosurg Psych* 1995; **59**: 38–44.

9. Comi G, Amadio S, Galardi G et al. Clinical and neurophysiological assessment of immunoglobulin therapy in five patients with multifocal motor neuropathy. *J Neurol Neurosurg Psych* 1994; **57** (suppl): 35–37.

10. Leger JM, Younes-Chennoufi AB, Chassande B et al. Human immunoglobulin treatment of multifocal motor neuropathy and polyneuropathy associated with monoclonal gammopathy. *J Neurol Neurosurg Psych* 1994; **57** (suppl): 46–49.

11. Saperstein DS, Amato AA, Wolfe GI et al. Multifocal acquired demyelinating sensory and motor neuropathy: the Lewis–Sumner Syndrome. *Muscle Nerve* 1999; **22**: 560–566.

12. Kaji R, Shibasaki H, Kimura J. Multifocal demyelinating motor neuropathy: cranial nerve involvement and immunoglobulin therapy. *Neurology* 1992; **42**: 506–509.

13. Lange DJ, Trojaberg W, Latov N et al. Multifocal motor neuropathy with conduction block: is it a distinct clinical entity? *Neurology* 1992; **42**: 497–505.

14. Rudge P, Ochoa J, Gilliatt RW. Acute peripheral nerve compression in the baboon. *J Neurol Sci* 1974; **23**: 403–420.

15. Saida K, Sumner AJ, Saida T et al. Antiserum-mediated demyelination: relationship between remyelination and functional recovery. *Ann Neurol* 1980; **8**: 12–24.

16. LaFontaine S, Rasminsky M, Saida T, Sumner AJ. Conduction block in rat myelinated fibres following acute exposure to anti-galactocerebroside serum. *J Physiol* 1982; **323**: 287–306.

17. Brown WF, Feasby TE. Conduction block and denervation in Guillain–Barre polyneuropathy. *Brain* 1984; **107**: 219–239.

18. Oh SJ, Kim DE, Kuruguolu HR. What is the best diagnostic index of conduction block and temporal dispersion? *Muscle Nerve* 1994; **17**: 489–493.

19. Rhee RK, England JD, Sumner AJ. Computer simulation of conduction block: effects produced by actual block verse interphase cancellation. *Ann Neurol* 1990; **28**: 146–159.

20. Chaudhry V, Cornblath DR, Griffin JW et al. Multifocal motor neuropathy: electrodiagnostic features. *Muscle Nerve* 1994; **17**: 198–205.

21. Katz JS, Wolfe GI, Bryan WW et al. Electrophysiologic findings in multifocal motor neuropathy. *Neurology* 1997; **48**: 700–707.

22. Pakiam AS, Parry GJ. Multifocal motor neuropathy without overt conduction block. *Muscle Nerve* 1998; **21**: 243–245.

23. Weimer LH, Grewal RP, Lange DJ. Electrophysiologic abnormalities other than conduction block in multifocal motor neuropathy. *Muscle Nerve* 1994; **9**: A1089.

24. Kaji R, Oka N, Tsuji T et al. Pathological findings at the site of conduction block in multifocal motor neuropathy. *Ann Neurol* 1993; **33**: 152–158.

25. Rapport MM, Donnenfield H, Brunner W et al. Ganglioside patterns in amyotrophic lateral sclerosis brain regions. *Ann Neurol* 1985; **18**: 60–67.

26. Ledeen R. Gangliosides of the neuron. *Trends Neurosci* 1985; **8**: 12–24.

27. Kaji R, Kimura J. Facts and fallacies on anti-GM1 antibodies: physiology of motor neuropathies. *Brain* 1999; **122**: 797–798.

28. Ogawa-Goto K, Funamoto N, Abe T et al. Different ceramide compositions of gangliosides between human motor and sensory nerves. *J Neurochem* 1990; **55**: 1486–1493.

29. Sheikh KA, Deerinck TJ, Ellisman MH, Griffin JW. The distribution of ganglioside-like moieties in peripheral nerves. *Brain* 1999; **122**: 449–460.

30. Takigawa T, Yasuda H, Kikkawa R et al. Antibodies against GM1 ganglioside affect K+ and Na+ currents in isolated rat myelinated nerve fibers. *Ann Neurol* 1995; **37**: 436–442.

31. Waxman SG. Sodium channel blockade by antibodies: a new mechanism of neurological disease? *Ann Neurol* 1995; **37**: 421–423.

32. Pestronk A, Choksi R. Multifocal motor neuropathy. Serum IgM anti-GM1 ganglioside antibodies in most patients detected using covalent linkage of GM1 to ELISA plates. *Neurology* 1997; **49**: 1289–1292.

33. Carpo M, Allaria S, Scarlato G, Nobile-Orazio E. Anti-GM1 IgM antibodies in multifocal motor neuropathy: slightly improved detection with covalink ELISA technique. *Neurology* (in press).

34. Van Schaik IN, Bossuyt PM, Brand A, Vermeulen M. Diagnostic value of GM1 antibodies in motor neuron disorders and neuropathies: a meta-analysis. *Neurology* 1995; **45**: 1570–1577.

35. Santoro M, Uncini A, Corbo M et al. Experimental conduction block induced by serum from a patient with anti-GM1 antibodies. *Ann Neurol* 1992; **31**: 385–390

36. Van den Berg LH, Franssen H, Van Doorn PA, Wokke JH. Intravenous immunoglobulin treatment in lower motor neuron disease associated with highly raised anti-GM1 antibodies. *J Neurol Neurosurg Psych* 1997; **63**: 674–677.

37. Azulay JP, Blin O, Pouget J et al. Intravenous immunoglobulin treatment in patients with motor neuron syndromes associated with anti-GM1 antibodies: a double-blind, placebo controlled study. *Neurology* 1994; **44**: 429–432.

38. Tsai CP, Lin KP, Liao KK et al. Immunosuppressive treatment in lower motor neuron syndrome with autoantibodies against GM1. *Eur Neurol* 1993; **33**: 446–449.

39. Pestronk A, Lopate G, Kornberg AJ et al. Distal lower motor neuron syndrome with high-titer serum IgM anti-GM1 antibodies: improvement following immunotherapy with monthly plasma exchange and intravenous cyclophosphamide. *Neurology* 1994; **44**: 2027–2031.

40. Van den Berg LH, Franssen H, Wokke JHJ. The long term effect of intravenous immunoglobulin treatment in multifocal motor neuropathy. *Brain* 1998; **121**: 421–428.

41. Van den Berg LH, Franssen H, Wokke JHJ. Improvement of multifocal motor neuropathy during long-term weekly treatment with human immunoglobulin. *Neurology* 1995; **45**: 987–988.

42. Van den Berg LH, Kerkhoff H, Oey PL et al. Treatment of multifocal motor neuropathy with high dose intravenous immunoglobulin: a double blind, placebo controlled study. *J Neurol Neurosurg Psych* 1995; **59**: 248–252.

43. Elliott JL, Pestronk A. Progression of multifocal motor neuropathy during apparently successful treatment with human immunoglobulin. *Neurology* 1994; **44**: 967–968.

44. Donaghy M, Mills KR, Boniface SJ et al. Pure motor demyelinating neuropathy: deterioration after steroid treatment and improvement with intravenous immunoglobulin. *J Neurol Neurosurg Psych* 1994; **57**: 778–783.

45. Azulay JP, Rihet P, Pouget J et al. Long term follow up of multifocal motor neuropathy with conduction block under treatment. *J Neurol Neurosurg Psych* 1997; **62**: 391–394.

46. Feldman EL, Bromberg MB, Albers JW, Pestronk A. Immunosuppressive treatment in multifocal motor neuropathy. *Ann Neurol* 1991; **30**: 397–401.

47. Van den Berg LH, Lokhorst H, Wokke JHJ. Pulsed high-dose dexamethasone is not effective in patients with multifocal motor neuropathy. *Neurology* 1997; **48**: 1135.

48. Pestronk A. Multifocal motor neuropathy: diagnosis and treatment. *Neurology* 1998; **51** (**suppl 5**): S22–S24.

49. Nobile-Orazio E, Meucci N, Barbieri S et al. High-dose intravenous immunoglobulin therapy in multifocal motor neuropathy. *Neurology* 1993; **43**: 537–544.

50. Oh SJ, Claussen GC, Kim DS. Motor and sensory demyelinating mononeuropathy multiplex (multifocal motor and sensory demyelinating neuropathy): a separate entity or a variant of chronic inflammatory demyelinating polyneuropathy. *J Periph Nerv Sys* 1997; **2**: 362–369.

51. Corse AM, Chaudhry V, Crawford TO et al. Sensory nerve pathology in multifocal motor neuropathy. *Ann Neurol* 1996; **39**: 319–325.

52. Parry GJ. Are multifocal motor neuropathy and Lewis–Sumner syndrome distinct nosologic entities? *Muscle Nerve* 1999; **22**: 557–559.

53. Lewis RA. Relationship of multifocal motor neuropathy and Lewis–Sumner syndrome. *Muscle Nerve* (in press).

54. Nikhar NJ, Lewis RA. Multifocal sensorimotor demyelinating neuropathy with persistent conduction block is distinct from multifocal motor neuropathy. *Neurology* 1998; **50 (suppl)**: A206.

55. Asbury AK, Aldredge H, Hershberg R, Fisher CM. Oculomotor palsy in diabetes mellitus: a clinico-pathological study. *Brain* 1970; **93**: 555–566.

56. Dreyfus PM, Hakim S, Adams RD. Diabetic ophthalmoplegia: report of case, with postmortem study and comments on vascular supply of human oculomotor nerve. *AMA Arch Neurol Psych* 1957; **77**: 337–349.

57. Kikta DG, Breuer AC, Wilbourn AJ. Thoracic root pain in diabetes: the spectrum of clinical and electromyographic findings. *Ann Neurol* 1982; **11**: 80–85.

58. Garland H. Diabetic amyotrophy. *Br Med J* 1955; **2**: 1287–1290.

59. Chokroverty S, Reyes MG, Rubino FA, Tonaki H. The syndrome of diabetic syndrome of diabetic amyotrophy. *Ann Neurol* 1977; **2**: 181–194.

60. Asbury AK. Proximal diabetic neuropathy. *Ann Neurol* 1977; **2**: 179–180.

61. Bradley WS, Chad D, Verghese JP et al. Painful lumbosacral plexopathy with elevated erythrocyte sedimentation rate: a treatable inflammatory syndrome. *Ann Neurol* 1984; **15**: 457–464.
62. Dyck PJB, Norrell J, Dyck PJ. Microscopic vasculitis in non-diabetic lumbosacral radiculoplexus neuropathy (LSRPN). *Neurology* 1999; **52** (suppl): A308.
63. Raff MC, Asbury AK. Ischemic mononeuropathy and mononeuropathy multiplex in diabetes mellitus. *New Engl J Med* 1968; **279**: 17–22.
64. Said G, Goulon-Goeau C, Lacroix C, Moulonguet A. Nerve biopsy findings in different patterns of proximal diabetic neuropathy. *Ann Neurol* 1994; **35**: 559–569.
65. Krendel DA, Costigan DA, Hopkins LC. Successful treatment of neuropathies in patients with diabetes mellitus. *Arch Neurol* 1995; **52**: 1053–1061.
66. Kelkar PM, Masood M, Parry GJ. Unique pathological findings in patients with proximal diabetic neuropathy (DPN). *Neurology* 1999; **52** (suppl): A309.
67. Simmons Z, Albers JW, Sima AA. Case-of-the-month: perineuritis presenting as mononeuritis multiplex. *Muscle Nerve* 1992; **15**: 630–635.
68. Sorenson EJ, Sima AAF, Blaivas M et al. Clinical features of perineuritis. *Muscle Nerve* 1997; **20**: 1153–1157.
69. Llewelyn JG, Thomas PK, King RH. Epineural microvasculitis in proximal diabetic neuropathy. *J Neurol* 1998; **245**: 159–165.
70. Krendel DA, Skehan ME. Patients with type I diabetes mellitus are predisposed to chronic inflammatory polyneuropathy. *Neurology* 1998; **50**: A333.
71. Krendel DA, Zacharias A, Skehan ME. Treatment of neuropathy associated with diabetes: an analysis of 55 patients. *J Neurol* 1997; **244**: S40–S41.
72. Stewart JD, McKelvey R, Durcan L et al. Chronic inflammatory demyelinating polyneuropathy (CIDP) in diabetics. *J Neurol Sci* 1996; **142**: 59–64.
73. Younger DS, Rosoklija G, Hays AP et al. Diabetic peripheral neuropathy: a clinicopathologic and immunohistochemical analysis of sural nerve biopsies. *Muscle Nerve* 1996; **19**: 722–727.
74. Pascoe MK, Low PA, Windebank AJ, Litchy WJ. Subacute diabetic proximal neuropathy. *Mayo Clin Proc* 1997; **72**: 1123–1132.
75. Jaradeh SS, Prieto TE, Lobeck LJ. Progressive polyradiculopathy in diabetes: correlation of variables and clinical outcome after immunotherapy. *J Neurol Neurosurg Psych* 1999; **67**: 607–612.

Chronic inflammatory demyelinating polyneuropathy

Pieter A van Doorn

3

> AIDP: acute immune-mediated demyelinating polyneuropathy; CIDP: chronic inflammatory demyelinating polyneuropathy; CSF: cerebrospinal fluid; GBS: Guillain–Barré syndrome; IVIG: intravenous immunoglobulin; MGUSP: monoclonal gammopathy of undetermined significance polyneuropathy; MMN: multifocal motor neuropathy; MP: methylprednisolone; PE: plasma exchange; SIDP: subacute inflammatory demyelinating polyneuropathy

Introduction

Chronic inflammatory demyelinating polyneuropathy (CIDP) is considered to be the chronic variety of the Guillain–Barré syndrome (GBS), an acute immune-mediated polyneuropathy.[1,2] In most cases, GBS is preceded by an infection in the 3 weeks prior to the onset of muscle weakness. In CIDP, a relapse or worsening of disease is frequently preceded by an infection. Most patients with GBS or CIDP develop considerable weakness and sensory disturbances due to dysfunction of peripheral nerves. It has been shown that several treatment options favour the outcome in both GBS and CIDP. Intravenous immunoglobulin (IVIG) treatment has already been administered with success from the early 1980s. Treatment trials later on showed efficacy of IVIG in both GBS[3,4] and CIDP (see below).

Diagnosis

CIDP and GBS differ mainly in onset, course and prognosis.

Duration of progressive weakness

Patients with GBS or the acute immune-mediated demyelinating polyneuropathy (AIDP) have progressive weakness for less than 4 weeks.[5] Most patients with CIDP have a progressive phase of weakness lasting 2 months at least.[6] In fact, these neuropathies are the poles of a spectrum, ranging from the acute variety of GBS on one side to a very slowly progressive CIDP on the other side. Patients with a progressive phase exceeding 4 weeks but less than 8 weeks are considered to have 'subacute' inflammatory demyelinating polyneuropathy (SIDP) (*Table 3.1*).[7]

The duration of progressive weakness allows the distinction between GBS and CIDP. Some patients with an initially rapid progressive phase of weakness resembling GBS then have a more gradual progression of their disease. These patients finally seem to have CIDP despite the acute onset of disease. It is good to realize that patients with a rapid progressive course with slow recovery still have GBS and do not shift towards CIDP, since the duration of progressive weakness makes the distinction between these disorders. Treatment of GBS needs to be administered within a short period, usually starting within the first 2 weeks after the onset of progressive weakness. In general, in CIDP there is no rapid progression of weakness. The course of CIDP may be gradual, with steps of

Table 3.1
Distinction between acute immune-mediated demyelinating polyneuropathy (AIDP), subacute inflammatory demyelinating polyneuropathy (SIDP) and chtonic inflammatory demyelinating polyneuropathy (CIDP).

Type of disease	Duration of progressive weakness
AIDP/GBS	<4 weeks
SIDP	4–8 weeks
CIDP	>8 weeks

progression, or may consist of spontaneous relapses and remissions. The fact that most CIDP patients need to be treated for a long period offers the possibility of switching between treatments or adding additional treatment. Especially because of the different treatments shown to be effective, it is important to make the distinction between GBS and CIDP (see below).

Clinical features

Patients with CIDP in general have symmetric weakness. A minority have predominant sensory disturbances. Other important findings are an increased level of CSF protein without cellular reaction and EMG findings compatible with demyelination. Criteria for CIDP have been published.[6,8] Recently new criteria were provided.[9] Practical diagnostic criteria for CIDP are summarized in *Table 3.2*.

Differential diagnosis

It is important to distinguish CIDP from several other disorders, especially since CIDP

Table 3.2
Practical diagnostic criteria for CIDP.

Clinical
1. Progressive symmetrical weakness of arms and legs for at least 2 months
2. Sensory disturbances generally less prominent; pain—if present—is unusually not prominent
3. Low or absent tendon reflexes
4. Sometimes cranial nerve palsies
5. Ventilator dependency is very unusual

Cerebrospinal fluid
1. Normal cell count; sometimes minor pleocytosis (<20/3 mononuclear cells/mm^3)
2. Total protein almost always elevated (often >1.0 g/l)

Nerve conduction studies
1. Delayed nerve conduction velocities
2. Increased distal latencies
3. Conduction blocks
4. Dispersion
5. Decreased excitability[10]

Important
Other causes of a chronic neuropathy must be ruled out or are very unlikely

Table 3.3
Important disorders in the differential diagnosis of CIDP.

1. Hereditary neuropathies (HMSN I, X-linked HMSN, HNLPP)
2. Paraproteinaemia (MGUSP, POEMS)
3. Intoxications (drugs, e.g. amiodarone)
4. Chronic idiopathic axonal neuropathy (CIAP)
5. Vasculitis (nonsystemic)
6. Multifocal motor neuropathy, especially in the chronic symmetric stage
7. Thyroid dysfunction
8. Remitting GBS
9. Subacute idiopathic demyelinating polyneuropathy (SIDP)

is a potentially treatable neuropathy. Important disorders in the differential diagnosis of CIDP are those that give rise to a demyelinating polyneuropathy. Patients with a chronic axonal neuropathy may also have some slowing of nerve conduction due to loss of nerves with rapid conduction properties. This may be a confusing finding, leading to a wrong diagnosis (*Table 3.3*).

Whether the presence of a serum monoclonal gammopathy rules out the diagnosis of CIDP is still a matter of debate. According to the research criteria of Cornblath et al, the presence of a monoclonal paraproteinaemia does not fit with the diagnosis of CIDP.[6] This may hold true in criteria for research purposes, but from a practical clinical point of view there is no consensus. There seems to be no doubt that this is the right decision in patients with a chronic demyelinating neuropathy with an IgM monoclonal protein, but patients over 50 years of age with an IgG-MGUS and otherwise typical signs and symptoms of CIDP can probably be treated in the same way as patients with CIDP in the absence of a monoclonal gammopathy.[11–14] In the author's series of over 70 patients who met the clinical and electrophysiological features of CIDP, about 7% had an IgG monoclonal gammopathy. There appeared to be no difference in response to treatment compared with those without an IgG monoclonal gammopathy.

Pathophysiology

Preceding infections

The pathogenesis of GBS and CIDP is possibly the same. About 70% of GBS patients had a preceding infection, most frequently with *Campylobacter jejuni*.[15,16]

CIDP is a long-lasting disorder and preceding infections are not studied as well as in GBS. In the author's series of CIDP patients it became clear that at least relapses were frequently associated with a preceding infection, once more indicating the relationship with GBS (unpublished results).

Antibodies

It is debatable whether CIDP is associated with a specific antibody response directed against neural antigens. Antibodies against a selected neuroblastoma cell line have been found in about 40% of patients with GBS and CIDP, compared with 5% in patients with other polyneuropathies.[17] Antibodies against various glycolipids (GM1, GD1b, GD1a, GT1b, GM2 and LM1) have been demonstrated in patients with CIDP but mostly in a small proportion of patients.[18] One group found that CIDP is not associated with antibodies to major glycolipids or myelin proteins.[19] Others described elevated titres of IgM antibodies against sulphated glucuronyl paragloboside (SGPG) and a relation with anti-GM1 antibodies.[20] Debate continues over how these antibodies may cause specific forms of disease.[21-23]

Impulse transmission and experimental studies

Studies on the pathophysiology of GBS and especially the Miller Fisher syndrome (a cranial nerve variant of GBS) have revealed evidence that serum of these patients can interfere with nerve impulse propagation. Studies using mouse phrenic nerve diaphragm preparation showed transmission failure after addition of serum containing GQ1b antibodies from MFS patients.[24] This effect seems to be complement-dependent.[25] Using patch clamp technique, it was shown that transmission failure could be achieved with serum from acute-stage GBS patients. Additional studies showed that this effect was IgG mediated and surprisingly was complement-independent and not related to the presence of detectable antibodies to GM1 or GQ1b.[26,27] Whether these effects can also be obtained using serum from patients with CIDP is not yet known.

An experimental study by Shy et al showed that heterozygous P0 knockout mice develop a neuropathy that resembles CIDP.[28] These mice developed a neuropathy with slowed motor nerve conduction, temporal dispersion and conduction block with histological signs of focal demyelination and inflammatory infiltrates. This suggests that at least in these mice, there may be an important role for myelin protein antigens such as P0.

What causes the difference between GBS and CIDP?

There is no evidence that there is a persisting antigenic stimulation in CIDP, or any indication that the level of antigenic stimulation differs between GBS and CIDP. Careful studies on preceding infections, further investigation of antibody production and T-cell-mediated responses to peripheral nerve antigens, combined with immunogenetic studies, may provide answers.

Treatment

Many uncontrolled studies and only a few controlled trials have been performed in CIDP. Controlled studies and the largest other series evaluating the effect of steroids and plasma exchange (PE) are discussed below. Clinical trials and other studies on the initial and long-term effects of intravenous immunoglobulin (IVIG) are discussed in more detail. The available data support thoughts that there are differences in treatment principles between GBS and CIDP (*Table 3.4*).

Steroids

Steroids are considered to be effective in patients with CIDP. It is, however, reported that improvement after prednisone was often not apparent over protracted periods.[29] A controlled trial in 28 patients treated with 120 mg prednisone every other day with tapering in 3 months, compared with no treatment, showed that prednisone caused a small but significant improvement.[30] The two largest retrospective studies reported improvement after corticosteroids in 49 of 76 (65%),[31] and in 56 of 59 (95%) CIDP patients.[8] The time lapse between initiation of prednisone treatment until onset of clinical improvement varied from 1–2 weeks up to 3.5 months.[32] Others reported that the mean time to the first signs of improvement was 1.9 (± 3.6) months and maximal improvement was reached no earlier than after 6.6 (± 5.4) months.[8] Although it was concluded that the majority of patients initially improved, relapses after discontinuation of steroids occurred in 70% of patients.[8] Additionally, it is well known that long-term treatment with corticosteroids can cause serious side-effects.

Table 3.4
Differences in treatment principles between GBS and CIDP.

GBS	Start treatment preferably within first 2 weeks after onset of disease
	One treatment course seems generally sufficient
CIDP	Long-term treatment necessary in most patients
	Possible to switch between treatments during the course of disease

Plasma exchange

Two plasma exchange (PE) trials in CIDP have been performed. In one study, 15 patients were treated with PE and 14 patients received a sham exchange.[33] The results were in favour of the PE-treated group. It appeared that improvement after PE was transient, since it began to fade 10–14 days after finishing the course of PE. The other study—in newly diagnosed, previously untreated CIDP patients—had a double-blind, sham-controlled, crossover design.[34] Eighteen previously untreated patients received PE for 4 weeks. After a wash-out period, the patients were crossed over. Three patients did not complete the trial; 15 patients could be analyzed. Twelve of these 15 patients (80%) had a major response to PE. Seven of the 12 patients (58%) relapsed 7–14 days after the last PE, but these patients could be stabilized with subsequent PE plus immunosuppressive drug therapy. There is no reported study that focuses on long-term treatment with PE. This is a drawback since long-term treatment seems to be inevitable in most patients with a CIDP. PE is expensive, it needs special equipment and good vascular access. These are important reasons favouring the choice of another proven effective treatment (steroids or IVIG) in patients with CIDP.

IVIG treatment

Initial phase

The first study of a group of CIDP patients treated with IVIG was published in 1985.[35] Since then, several uncontrolled studies claimed that 20–100% of CIDP patients improved after IVIG treatment (for review see Van Doorn[36]). The initial dosage that is generally used is 2.0 g/kg divided over 2–5 days. In a retrospective study involving 52 CIDP patients, it was found that 32 patients (62%) improved after IVIG. Twenty-one patients (40%) needed intermittent IVIG infusions to maintain clinical improvement, suggesting that improvement—at least in these patients—was caused by IVIG treatment.[11] In two of the 32 patients, there was a brief improvement and subsequent IVIG infusions had no effect.

In a retrospective study, the following variables were significantly associated with a high chance for improvement after IVIG treatment: disease duration of less than 1 year, progression of weakness until treatment, no discrepancy in weakness between arms and legs, areflexia of the arms, and slowed motor nerve conduction velocity of the median nerve.[11] It was calculated that the chance of improvement after IVIG was over 90% if these five factors were present. These factors together suggest that CIDP patients with active disease and weakness both in arms and legs are most likely to improve after IVIG.

Placebo-controlled trials

Three double-blind placebo-controlled trials have been published.[37–39] In the first crossover trial it was shown that all seven CIDP patients improved after IVIG and none of the patients responded after placebo treatment.[37] Improvement after IVIG was always observed within 1 week after the start of treatment. The time lapse from the end of trial treatment to deterioration was significantly longer after treatment with IVIG (mean 6.4 weeks) than after placebo treatment (mean 1.3 weeks). Surprisingly, another trial could not demonstrate the efficacy of IVIG treatment in a double-blind, placebo-controlled study in 28 patients with a clinical diagnosis of CIDP who were not treated with IVIG previously.[38] One reason for this unexpected result could be the observation that three patients with a slowly progressive deterioration before the start of trial treatment had an unexpected rapid and dramatic clinical improvement within days after the start of placebo treatment suggesting rapid spontaneous improvement. Another explanation for the negative results may be the skewed deviation of CIDP patients within the treatment groups: as many as 10 of 13 patients in the placebo group and only 6 out of 15 patients in the IVIG treatment group fulfilled the five criteria that were associated with improvement after IVIG treatment.[11] These observations indicate that only a subgroup of patients with a CIDP seem to respond to IVIG treatment. In the third trial, 30 patients with CIDP were examined in a double-blind, placebo-controlled, crossover trial. After IVIG, 10 of the 17 chronic progressive patients (60%) and 9 of the 13 relapsing patients (69%) clinically improved ($p \leq 0.002$).[39] Some improvement was also seen in five patients after placebo treatment; this may indicate that the course of disease may fluctuate more than generally expected.

Long-term treatment

No trial has yet evaluated the effect of IVIG over a long period. The proportion of patients who improve after IVIG depends on selection criteria (see above) and seems to vary between 60% and 90%. Only a small proportion of patients with chronic progressive disease have a long-lasting remission after a single course of IVIG treatment. In the author's series of over 70 patients treated with IVIG almost all patients finally reached clinical remission. Around 50% of the patients who initially improved needed intermittent IVIG treatment for over 3.5 years. A small minority of patients even needed intermittent IVIG for a period exceeding 10 years, indicating that IVIG seems to suppress disease activity rather than induce remission.[40] IVIG treatment appeared to be relatively safe, as no serious side-effects were observed. However, this treatment is extremely expensive, an incentive to add additional treatment or to switch to another treatment somewhat earlier during the course of disease.

Treatment schedule

When treating CIDP patients with IVIG, the author's practice is to start with IVIG 2 g/kg for 2–5 days. If the patient improves after these infusions, this becomes clinically obvious 7–9 days after the start of treatment. Only if improvement wanes, IVIG treatment 0.4 g/kg per day is repeated for 1–3 days. If the patient later deteriorates again, intermittent IVIG is given once every 2–4 weeks. The individual treatment frequency is dependent on the clinical signs and symptoms of disease activity.[11,36,41]

Comparison of treatment with steroids, PE or IVIG

Several uncontrolled studies have included CIDP patients who were treated with PE, steroids or other immunosuppressive treatments prior to or after failure of IVIG treatment. These studies show that some CIDP patients may improve after steroids, PE or IVIG, while other patients improve only after one particular treatment.[11,36,42] This means that it is generally worth while trying another treatment if prednisone, PE or IVIG fails.

There is only one controlled study comparing PE (five sessions) with IVIG (in total 1.8 g/kg).[43] In this crossover study 20 patients were randomized. Only 13 received both treatments, whereas four did not worsen sufficiently to receive the second treatment; three patients left the study for various reasons. With both treatment schedules, statistical significant improvement occurred for: overall neurological disability score, muscle weakness, and compound muscle action potentials (CMAP) ($p < 0.001$–0.006). Improvement after IVIG was comparable to the effect of PE. The authors suggest that IVIG may be the preferable initial treatment in many patients.

The cost of treatment is important. IVIG and PE are both expensive. To compare the costs of IVIG and PE, one has to take into account also the costs for PE personnel, equipment and other logistics. In the Netherlands, and also in the USA, the costs for five PE sessions or an IVIG course with in total 2 g/kg seem to be more or less equal.[44] Corticosteroids on the other hand are cheap, but the complications can be severe and expensive as well. Because of the potential serious side-effects of prednisone, especially in children, treatment is started with IVIG as soon as the patient has reached a degree of muscular weakness that significantly interferes with life style or prevents an independent existence. The effectiveness, advantages and disadvantages of PE, steroids and IVIG treatment are summarized in *Table 3.5*.

Pilot studies

An open study in 10 patients with CIDP suggests that treatment with pulsed high-dose

Table 3.5
Treatment of CIDP.

Treatment	Effect	Potential side-effects	Availability	Direct cost
Prednisone	+	Severe	Very good	Low
Plasma exchange	+	Minor	Rather good	High
IVIG	+	Minor/none	Good	High

dexamethasone is effective.[45] It is suggested that this regimen may have advantages compared with conventional prednisone treatment, since it may induce remissions more adequately. A controlled trial has not yet been performed. Small or noncontrolled studies indicate that cyclosporin is effective in otherwise treatment-resistant CIDP patients.[46] Recent studies report improvement of CIDP following interferon alfa-2a,[47] and interferon beta-1a.[48] At present these treatments should be regarded only as options when standard treatment fails.

Mechanism of action of IVIG

It is known from studies on various autoimmune diseases that IVIG can intervene at various levels.[49-51] Studies on the mechanism of IVIG in CIDP are limited. In vitro studies showed that IVIG contains antiidiotypic antibodies that recognize a cross-reactive idiotype on antineuroblastoma cell line antibodies. These antibodies are present in serum of about 40% of patients with GBS or CIDP. F(ab)$_2$ antibodies present in serum from recovered GBS patients can inhibit antineuroblastoma cell line antibody activity in serum from patients with CIDP or with active GBS.[14,52-54] It is, however, not proved that the various antibodies including anti-neuroblastoma cell line antibodies present in GBS and in CIDP patients have a direct pathogenic role in the process of disease. Whether a large pool of donors is essential for improvement of GBS or CIDP is questionable since it was observed that improvement from CIDP can also occur after intermittent infusion of fresh frozen plasma obtained from a limited number (20–28) of donors.[35] A recent case report suggests that the mechanism of IVIG in CIDP is not mainly mediated by aspecific Fc interaction.[55] The mechanism of action of IVIG in patients with GBS or CIDP is far from clarified. In vitro studies indicate that V region-dependent interaction plays a role in the regulation of GBS and CIDP.[53] Recent studies suggest that IVIG interferes with anti-GM1 antibodies either by direct bindings[56] or by inhibition of binding to its target antigen.[57]

Conclusion

It has been shown that prednisone treatment is effective in CIDP.[30] PE was shown to be effective in two studies.[33,34] In two placebo-controlled studies it was found that IVIG is effective.[37,39] One study did not show a difference in treatment effect between PE and IVIG.[43] One of the advantages of IVIG is its good availability and rapid clinical effect (within 9 days after onset of treatment). A great disadvantage is its price. The percentage of patients improving after prednisone, PE or IVIG seems to be around 70–80%, but appears—at least when treated with IVIG—to be dependent on the selection of patients. Some patients may need a combination of treatments during the course of disease. The conducted trials only investigated the initial effect of treatment. Additional studies are necessary to obtain more information on the clinical effect and side-effects of treatment during the long-term course of the disease.

References

1. Dyck PJ, Prineas J, Pollard JD. Chronic inflammatory demyelinating polyneuropathy. In: Dyck and Thomas, eds. *Peripheral Neuropathy,* 3rd edition. Philadelphia: Saunders, 1993, 1498–1518.

2. Hahn AF. Guillain–Barré syndrome. *Lancet* 1998; **352**: 635–641.

3. Van der Meché FGA, Schmitz PIM, Dutch Guillain–Barré Study Group. A randomized trial comparing intravenous immune globulin and plasma exchange in Guillain–Barré syndrome. *New Engl J Med* 1992; **326**: 1123–1129.

4. Plasma exchange/Sandoglobulin Guillain–Barré syndrome trial group. Randomised trial of plasma exchange, intravenous immunoglobulin, and combined treatments in Guillain–Barré syndrome. *Lancet* 1997; **349**: 225–230.

5. Asbury AK, Cornblath DR. Assessment of current diagnostic criteria for Guillain–Barré syndrome. *Ann Neurol* 1990; **27** (**suppl**): S21–S24.

6. Cornblath DR, Asbury AK, Albers JW et al. Research criteria for diagnosis of chronic inflammatory demyelinating polyneuropathy (CIDP). *Neurology* 1991; **41**: 617–618.

7. Hughes RAC, Sanders E, Hall S et al. Subacute idiopathic demyelinating polyradiculoneuropathy. *Arch Neurol* 1992; **49**: 612–616.

8. Barohn RJ, Kissel JT, Warmolts et al. Chronic inflammatory demyelinating polyradiculoneuropathy, clinical characteristics, course and recommendations for diagnostic criteria. *Arch Neurol* 1989; **14**: 878–884.

9. Franssen H, Vermeulen M, Jennekens FGI. Chronic inflammatory neuropathies. In: Hemery AEH, ed. *Diagnostic Criteria for Neuromuscular Disorders,* 2nd edition. London: Royal Society of Medicine Press, 1997, 53–59.

10. Meulstee J, Darbas A, van Doorn PA et al. Decreased electrical excitability of peripheral

nerves in demyelinating polyneuropathies. *J Neurol Neurosurg Psych* 1997; **62**: 398–400.

11. Van Doorn PA, Vermeulen M, Brand A et al. Intravenous immunoglobulin treatment in patients with chronic inflammatory demyelinating polyneuropathy. Clinical and laboratory characteristics associated with improvement. *Arch Neurol* 1991; **48**: 217–220.

12. Simmons Z, Albers JW, Bromberg M et al. Longterm follow-up of patients with CIDP, with and without monoclonal gammopathy. *Brain* 1995; **118**: 359–368.

13. Van Doorn PA, Brand A, Vermeulen M. Anti-neuroblastoma cell line antibodies in inflammatory demyelinating polyneuropathy: inhibition in vitro and in vivo by IV immunoglobulin. *Neurology* 1988; **38**: 1592–1595.

14. Ilyas AA, Mithen FA, Dalakas MC et al. Antibodies to acidic glycolipids in Guillain–Barré syndrome and chronic inflammatory demyelinating polyneuropathy. *J Neurol Sci* 1992; **107**: 111–121.

15. Rees JH, Soudain SE, Gregson NA et al. A prospective case control study to investigate the relationship between *Campylobacter jejuni* infection and Guillain–Barré syndrome. *New Engl J Med* 1995; **333**: 1374–1379.

16. Jacobs BC, Rothbarth P, van der Meché FGA et al. The spectrum of antecedent infections in Guillain–Barré syndrome: a case-control study. *Neurology* 1998; **51**: 1110–1115.

17. Dyck PJ. Intravenous immunoglobulin in chronic inflammatory demyelinating polyradiculoneuropathy and in neuropathy associated with IgM monoclonal gammopathy of unknown significance. *Neurology* 1990; **40**: 327–328.

18. Dyck PJ, Low PA, Windebank AJ et al. Plasma exchange in polyneuropathy associated with monoclonal gammopathy of undetermined significance. *New Engl J Med* 1991; **325**: 1482–1486.

19. Melendez-Vasquez C, Redford J, Choudhary PP et al. Immunological investigation of chronic inflammatory demyelinating polyradiculoneuropathy. *J Neuroimmunol* 1997; **73**: 124–134.

20. Yuki N, Tagawa Y, Handa S. Autoantibodies to peripheral nerve glycosphingolipids SPG, SLPG, and SGPG in Guillain–Barré syndrome and chronic inflammatory demyelinating polyneuropathy. *J Neuroimmunol* 1996; **70**: 1–6.

21. Willison HJ, O'Hanlon G, Paterson G et al. Mechanism of action of anti-GM1 and anti-GQ1b ganglioside antibodies in Guillain–Barré syndrome. *J Infect Dis* 1997; **176(Suppl 2)**: S144–S149.

22. Feasby TE, Hughes RAC. Campylobacter jejuni, anti-ganglioside antibodies and Guillain–Barré syndrome. *Neurology* 1998; **51**: 334–342.

23. Hartung HP, van der Meche FGA, Pollard JD. Guillain–Barré syndrome, CIDP and other chronic immune-mediated neuropathies. *Curr Opin Neurol* 1998; **11**: 497–513.

24. Roberts M, Willison HJ, Vincent A et al. Serum factor in Miller Fisher variant of Guillain–Barré syndrome and neurotransmitter release. *Lancet* 1994; **343**: 454–455.

25. Plomp JJ, Molenaar PC, O'Hanlon GH et al. Anti-GQ1b antibodies from patients with Miller Fisher anti-GQ1b antibodies; alpha-laterotoxin-like effects on motor end plates. *Ann Neurol* 1999; **45**: 189–199.

26. Buchwald B, Toyka KV, Zielasek J et al.

Neuromuscular blockade by IgG antibodies with Guillain–Barré syndrome: a macro-patch-clamp study. *Ann Neurol* 1998; **44:** 913–922.

27. Buchwald B, Weishaupt A, Toyka KV, Dudel J. Pre- and postsynaptic blockade of neuromuscular transmission by Miller-Fisher syndrome IgG at mouse motor nerve terminals. *Eur J Neurosci* 1998; **10:** 281–290.

28. Shy ME, Arroyo E, Sladky J et al. Heterozygous P0 knockout mice develop a peripheral neuropathy that resembles chronic inflammatory demyelinating polyneuropathy (CIDP). *J Neuropathol Exp Neurol* 1997; **56:** 811–821.

29. Dyck PJ, Lais AC, Ohta M et al. Chronic inflammatory polyradiculoneuropathy. *Mayo Clin Proc* 1975; **50:** 621–637.

30. Dyck PJ, O'Brien PC, Oviatt KF et al. Prednisone improves chronic inflammatory demyelinating polyradiculopathy more than no treatment. *Ann Neurol* 1982; **11:** 136–141.

31. McCombe PA, Pollard JD, McLeod JG. Chronic inflammatory demyelinating polyradiculoneuropathy. A clinical and electrophysiological study of 92 cases. *Brain* 1987; **110:** 1617–1630.

32. De Vivo DC, Engel WK. Remarkable recovery of a steroid-responsive recurrent polyneuropathy. *J Neurol Neurosurg Psych* 1970; **33:** 62–69.

33. Dyck PJ, Daube J, O'Brien PC et al. Plasma exchange in chronic inflammatory demyelinating polyradiculoneuropathy. *New Engl J Med* 1986; **314:** 461–465.

34. Hahn AF, Bolton CF, Pillay N et al. Plasma-exchange therapy in chronic inflammatory demyelinating polyneuropathy. A double-blind, sham-controlled, cross-over study. *Brain* 1996; **119:** 1055–1066.

35. Vermeulen M, van der Meché FGA, Speelman JD et al. Plasma and gamma-globulin infusion in chronic inflammatory demyelinating polyneuropathy. *J Neurol Sci* 1985; **70:** 317–326.

36. Van Doorn PA. Intravenous immunoglobulin treatment in patients with chronic inflammatory demyelinating polyneuropathy. *J Neurol Neurosurg Psych* 1994; **57 (suppl):** 38–42.

37. Van Doorn PA, Brand A, Strengers PFW et al. High-dose intravenous immunoglobulin treatment in chronic inflammatory demyelinating polyneuropathy. A double-blind placebo-controlled crossover study. *Neurology* 1990; **40:** 209–212.

38. Vermeulen M, Van Doorn PA, Brand A et al. Intravenous immunoglobulin treatment in patients with chronic inflammatory demyelinating polyneuropathy: a double-blind, placebo controlled study. *J Neurol Neurosurg Psych* 1993; **56:** 36–39.

39. Hahn AF, Bolton CF, Zochodne D, Faesby TE. Intravenous immunoglobulin treatment in chronic inflammatory demyelinating polyneuropathy. A double-blind, placebo controlled, cross-over study. *Brain* 1996; **119:** 1067–1077.

40. Van Doorn P, van Burken M, Vermeulen M et al. Long-term IV immunoglobulin (IVIg) treatment in patients with chronic inflammatory demyelinating polyneuropathy (CIDP). *J Neurol* 1996; **243 (suppl 2):** S33.

41. Van der Meché FGA, Van Doorn PA. Guillain–Barré syndrome and chronic inflammatory demyelinating polyneuropathy: immune mechanisms and update on current therapies. *Ann Neurol* 1995; **37 (S1):** S14–S31.

42. Nemni R, Amadio S, Fazio R et al.

Intravenous immunoglobulin treatment in patients with chronic inflammatory demyelinating neuropathy not responsive to other treatments. *J Neurol Neurosurg Psych* 1994; **57** (suppl): 43–45.

43. Dyck PJ, Litchy WJ, Kratz KM et al. A plasma exchange versus immune globulin infusion trial in chronic inflammatory demyelinating polyradiculoneuropathy. *Ann Neurol* 1994; **36**: 838–845.

44. Thornton CA, Griggs RC. Plasma-exchange and intravenous immunoglobulin treatment of neuromuscular disease. *Ann Neurol* 1994; **35**: 260–268.

45. Molenaar DSM, van Doorn PA, Vermeulen M. Pulsed high dose dexemethasone treatment in chronic inflammatory demyelinating polyneuropathy. Pilot study. *J Neurol Neurosurg Psych* 1997; **62**: 388–390.

46. Barnet MH, Polard JD, Davies L, McLeod JG. Cyclosporin A in resistant chronic inflammatory demyelinating polyradiculoneuropathy. *Muscle Nerve* 1998; **21**: 454–460.

47. Mahattanakul W, Crawford TO, Griffin JW et al. Treatment of chronic inflammatory demyelinating polyneuropathy with cyclosporin-A. *J Neurol Neurosurg Psych* 1996; **60**: 185–187.

48. Martina ISJ, Van Doorn PA, Meulstee J et al. Improvement of muscle strength in patients with chronic motor neuropathies treated with interferon-β (Rebif). *J Neurol Neurosurg Psych* 1999; **66**: 197–201.

49. Dwyer JM. Manipulating the immune system with immune globulin. *New Engl J Med* 1992; **326**: 107–116.

50. Hurez V, Kaveri SV, Kazatchkine MD. Normal polyspecific immunoglobulin G (IVIg) in the treatment of autoimmune diseases. *J Autoimmunity* 1993; **6**: 675–681.

51. Dalakas MC. Mechanism of action of intravenous immunoglobulin and therapeutic considerations in the treatment of autoimmune neurologic diseases. *Neurology* 1998; **51**: S2–S8.

52. Lundkvist I, Van Doorn PA, Vermeulen M et al. Regulation of autoantibodies in inflammatory demyelinating polyneuropathy: spontaneous and therapeutic. *Immunol Rev* 1989; **110**: 105–117.

53. Lundkvist I, Van Doorn PA, Vermeulen M et al. Spontaneous recovery from the Guillain–Barré syndrome is associated with anti-idiotypic antibodies recognizing a cross-reactive idiotype on anti-neuroblastoma cell line antibodies. *Clin Immunol Immunopathol* 1993; **67**: 192–198.

54. Van Doorn PA, Rossi F, Brand A et al. On the mechanism of high-dose intravenous immunoglobulin treatment of patients with chronic inflammatory demyelinating polyneuropathy. *J Neuroimmunol* 1990; **29**: 57–64.

55. Vermeulen M, Van Schaik IN. Anti-D immunoglobulin treatment in chronic inflammatory demyelinating polyneuropathy. *J Neurol Neurosurg Psych* 1995; **58**: 383–384.

56. Yuki N, Miyagi F. Possible mechanism of intravenous immunoglobulin treatment on anti-GM1 antibody-mediated neuropathies. *J Neurol Sci* 1996; **139**: 160–162.

57. Malik U, Oleksowicz L, Latov N, Cardo LJ. Intravenous gamma-globulin inhibits binding of anti-GM1 to its target antigen. *Ann Neurol* 1996; **39**: 136–139.

Prognostic factors in chronic inflammatory demyelinating polyneuropathy

Gérard Said

> CIDP: chronic inflammatory demyelinative polyneuropathy; CSF: cerebrospinal fluid

Chronic inflammatory demyelinative polyneuropathy (CIDP) is an acquired peripheral neuropathy with an onset period extending over more than 2 months. Based on a presumed immune-mediated mechanism, treatment with high doses of intravenous immunoglobulins (IVIG) is widely used in this setting. However, the response to treatments, whether IVIG, plasma exchange, corticosteroids or immunosuppressive drugs, is always difficult to predict. In the series of patients studied by Gorson et al[1] two-thirds of the patients with idiopathic CIDP responded to treatment with IVIG, plasma exchanges or corticosteroids. In a series of 83 patients assessed on average 6 years after the first manifestations of idiopathic CIDP, 24% of the patients failed to respond to any treatment after partial positive response during several years. Nine patients died from progression of the neurological deficit.[2] Thus, CIDP is a potentialy life-threatening condition, even though 47% of these patients remained in a stable condition. Identification of factors relevant to the outcome of this syndrome would therefore be important to adjust therapy.

From a clinicopathological point of view, CIDP is primarily a demyelinative neuropathy following a chronic progressive or a relapsing course, and often a secondary progressive course, after years of relapses and remissions. The demyelinative lesions are usually widespread and affect spinal roots, plexuses and peripheral nerves. Demyelination is typically mediated by macrophages, especially during the onset and relapses. Demyelination is associated with inflammatory infiltrates, proliferation of Schwann cells and a variable proportion of fibres undergoing axonal degeneration. However, these features are inconstantly found in biopsy specimens of patients with CIDP (Figs 4.1–4.3). In a study of 95 nerve biopsies of patients with CIDP, endoneurial cellularity was slightly increased in 18 nerve samples, with only four specimens showing conspicuous inflammatory infiltrates. In all cases the inflammatory infiltration was made of mononuclear cells and predominated around endoneurial blood vessels. In the four specimens with marked inflammatory infiltration, immunolabelling showed a mixture of CD4 and CD8 T lymphocytes, macrophages and a few B cells. Onion bulb formations due to accumulation of concentric Schwann cell processes resulting from repeated demyelination/remyelination, were present in 17 nerve specimens. The fate of axons is important to consider in this condition. In this series, the density of myelinated nerve fibres in biopsy specimens was below 50% of control values in 47% of the patients, and was less than 25% of control values in 25% of the patients. Thus in addition to primary demyelination, axons are often involved in CIDP. A recent study by Nagamatsu et al[3] of sural nerve biopsy in 71 patients with CIDP, and motor neuron pathology of postmortem examination of spinal cords of nine patients who died of CIDP, clearly confirms the importance of axonal and neuronal involvement in this setting. In Nagamatsu's study, the overall decreases of myelinated fibre density was 65.4% of control values. Thus axonal lesions are an important prognostic factor to consider in chronic demyelinative neuropathies, since recovery from axonal lesions takes much more time than recovery from demyelination and is often only partial.

In this respect it is important to recall that in demyelinating disorders that affect both the central and the peripheral nervous systems the neurological deficit results from impairment of axonal function, which can itself be the consequence of axonal degeneration or of conduction blocks. Acute demyelination can induce conduction blocks responsible for distal deficit. For technical reasons, conduction blocks are detected on motor

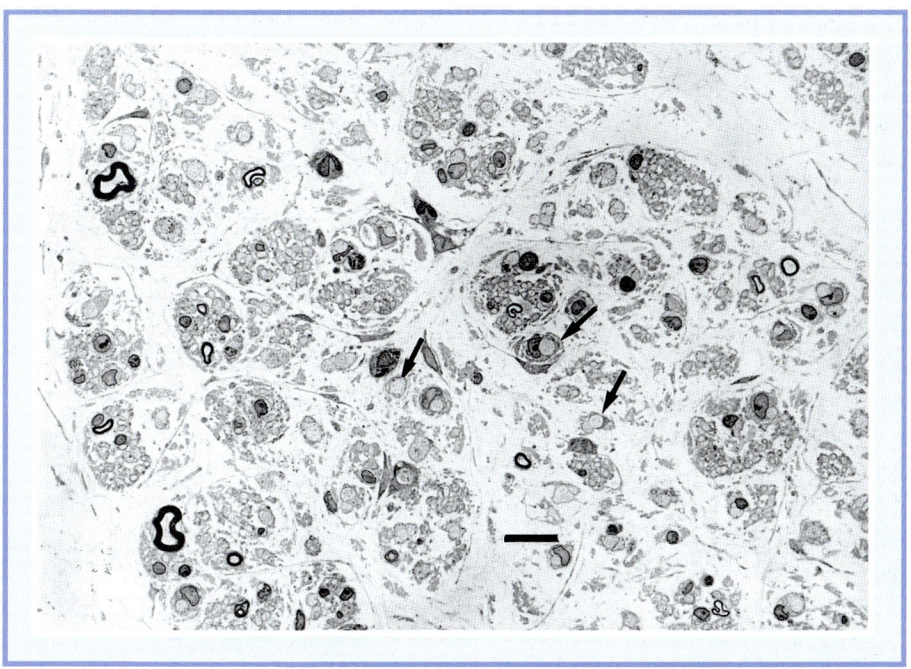

Figure 4.1
One micrometre thick plastic section of the superficial radial nerve of a 44-year-old woman who complained of oral paresthesia and pains in the hands. Neurological examination showed only questionable 'glove and stocking' hypoaesthesia. Strength was normal. Note the decreased density of nerve fibres (980 myelinated fibres per mm^2; N: 8000 myelinated fibres per mm^2), most of them demyelinated (arrows). There was no inflammatory infiltrate in this case. Scale bar 10 μm.

nerves only in practice. They are routinely found in peripheral nerves in Guillain–Barré syndrome or in CIDP. In experimental models, reversion of conduction blocks with subsequent functional recovery occurs within a few days after induction of acute demyelination by subperineurial injection of proteases.[4] Functional recovery and disappearance of conduction blocks are closely related to remyelination. Within 3–4 weeks after acute monophasic demyelination, muscle strength has returned to normal, as the conduction block has disappeared with remyelination of the demyelinated nerve segment. This pattern of lesions can be antibody-mediated, cell-mediated, or occur as

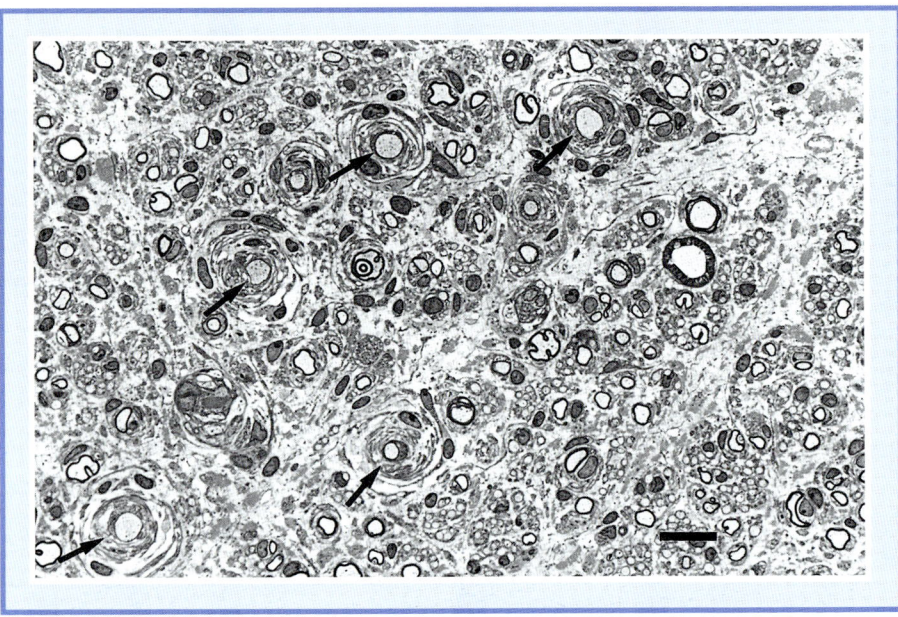

Figure 4.2
Sural nerve biopsy specimen of a patient with CIDP. Several onion bulb formations are visible around demyelinated axons (arrowed). The axon density is relatively preserved in this case. Scale bar 10 μm.

a result of a bystander effect due to release of products of macrophage activation in the context of a delayed hypersensitivity reaction. Spinal roots are predominantly affected in virtually all cases, but nerve trunks and terminal nerve endings can be affected too. When neurological deficit is predominantly or exclusively due to conduction blocks, spontaneous or treatment-induced improvement can occur within a few weeks, as observed in patients with Guillain–Barré syndrome. Unfortunately, axonal lesions are often associated with primary demyelination, and axonal regeneration by sprouting of the proximal stump is a slow process, often leading to a delayed and often partial recovery.

This phenomenon is particularly evident in severe lesions of spinal roots and proximal nerve trunks in patients dying of Guillain-Barré syndrome.[5–7] The axonal lesions occurring in the course of demyelinative neuropathy have been attributed to a

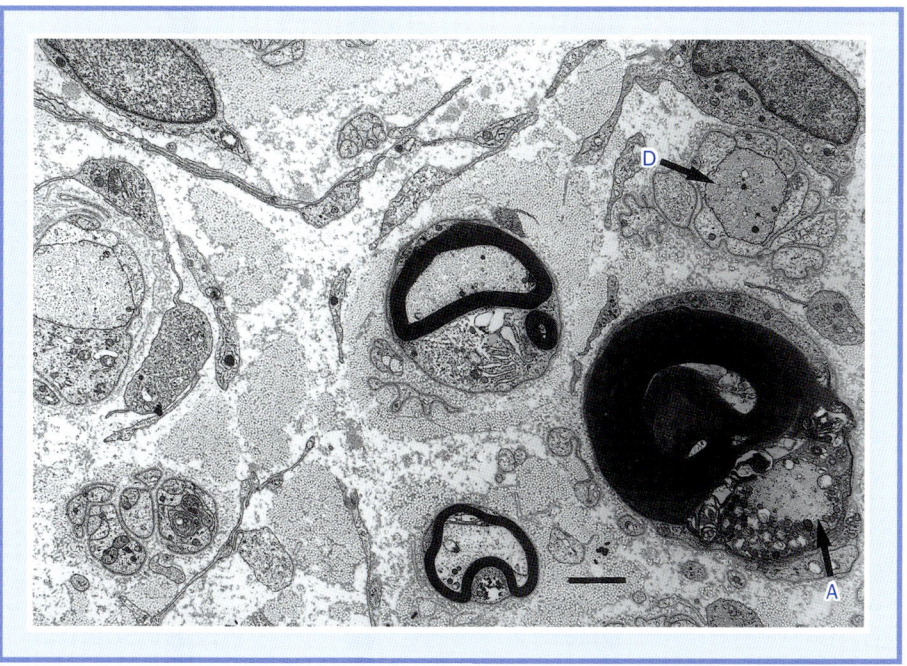

Figure 4.3
Electron micrograph of a sural nerve biopsy of a patient with progressive idiopathic CIDP. Note the presence of demyelinated fibres (D) and of a fibre with a damaged axon (A). Scale bar 2 μm.

bystander effect in inflammatory foci,[8,9] to immune attack directed toward epitopes on the axon[6] or to increased endoneurial pressure.[7] It is thus obvious that in demyelinating disorders of the peripheral and of the central nervous systems, the long-term prognosis depends more on the amplitude of axonal loss, as in multiple sclerosis, than on demyelination.

In previous studies clinical and electrophysiological prognostic factors have been evaluated. The following items were associated with a high probability of improvement: disease duration of less than 1 year, progression of weakness until treatment, absence of discrepancy in weakness between arms and legs, areflexia of the arms, and slowing of motor conduction velocities of the median nerve.[10] Another important problem encountered in evaluating the effects of treatments in CIDP, as in many neurological conditions, is related to the difficulty of quantifying sensory and motor impairment. In spite of relatively strict criteria applied to define CIDP, the clinical presentation, the course, the mixture of motor and sensory deficits, and the variable distribution of deficits make quantitative evaluation of neurological impairment very difficult.[11,12]

The prognostic factors that could be used in therapeutic decision-making were tested by comparing the main clinical and pathological findings in a series of 100 patients with CIDP of unknown origin investigated in the author's centre from 1979 to 1994, with the functional score assessed 6 years later on average. The criteria for CIDP for inclusion of patients were the following:

(a) symptomatic motor and/or sensory neuropathy of unknown origin affecting more than one limb;
(b) onset of neurological deficit extending over 2 months or more;
(c) electrophysiological and/or morphological features of demyelination;
(d) no detectable cause of neuropathy.

Patients with monoclonal gammopathy associated with chronic demyelinating polyneuropathy were excluded. Monoclonal gammopathy could be detected either at the initial examination or during follow-up. Infection with human immunodeficiency virus, and hereditary, metabolic or paraneoplastic disorders, were also excluded by appropriate investigations. This restricted the evaluation to patients with idiopathic CIDP.

Functional capability, based on a modified Norris score, was compared with the mode of onset, age of patients, the relapsing–remitting or progressive course of the disease and the cerebrospinal fluid (CSF) protein content. Ninety-five patients in this series also had a peripheral nerve biopsy of a sensory nerve in an affected territory for diagnostic confirmation, assessment of axon loss and evaluation of the activity of the neuropathy by incidence of fibres undergoing axonal degeneration or segmental demyelination. Morphological data allowed the comparison of the functional score of the patients with the different pathological components of CIDP.

The following features were compared with the functional disability score: age of patients less than 30 years and more than 60 years; pains at onset of the neuropathy; precession of the neuropathy by an infectious event; motor deficit at onset; relapsing or progressive course; high CSF protein; nerve biopsy findings including axonal loss, inflammatory infiltration, active demyelination and onion bulb formation. Axonal loss as a prognostic factor was calculated as the regression coefficient of axonal loss on functional capacity.

Seventy-four per cent of patients had a typical demyelinating pattern on electrophysiological tests; 14% had only one criterion of demyelination on nerve conduction studies. Fourteen per cent had nerve conduction blocks. No isolated or predominant axonal electrophysiological pattern was found, but there was a poor correlation between loss or microvolted sural nerve sensory action potential and relative preservation of fibre density in patients with CIDP.

Data from 83 patients were collected 6 years on average after the first manifestations of neuropathy. Eight patients (10%) with relapsing forms were in remission, and six had relapsed at the time of evaluation, giving a different functional score. At evaluation, 38 patients were able to work and 18 had retired without major disability. The outcome was good in 56% of the patients. Fourteen of the 83 patients died (17%), including nine who died as a result of progression of the neurological deficit to quadriplegia and respiratory and swallowing difficulty. Four patients died from an unknown cause, and one from pulmonary embolism. The mean age of the patients who died was 67 years compared with 49 years in the cohort. Of the others, 5 were bedridden, 6 had a severe handicap, 11 a mild handicap, and 23 a moderate handicap, while 24 were fully autonomous. Relapsing forms carried a better prognosis than progressive forms, in keeping with Hahn's findings that patients with acutely relapsing CIDP were likely to respond to IVIG treatment.[11] In contrast, Van Doorn et al[10] found no correlation between disease course and response to treatment. Twenty patients (24%), including the nine patients who died as a consequence of neurological deficit, resisted all treatments, after having partially responded for a few years.

A younger age at onset correlated with a better outcome in this series: patients under 30 years of age had moderate disability ($p < 0.05$), and no death occurred in this age group. Pains at onset and infectious events prior to the onset of the neuropathy were also associated with a better prognosis ($p < 0.05$). Conversely, central nervous system manifestations, which were associated with CIDP in five patients, were associated with a poorer outcome ($p < 0.05$), as was the presence of four-limb weakness at the onset ($p < 0.05$). Increased CSF protein content and severe demyelinating features on electrodiagnostic testing tended to be more frequent in patients with a poor outcome, but did not reach significance. Axon loss correlated positively with a poorer outcome ($p < 0.0001$). Active demyelination affected 60% of the nerve fibres in bedridden patients compared with 21% in autonomous patients ($p < 0.05$). Onion bulb formations were more common in patients with severe neuropathy, but the results were not significant ($p = 0.08$).

On several occasions the amplitude of the

sensory nerve action potentials did not fit well with morphological findings. In this setting, nerve biopsy may reveal relative preservation of the density of myelinated axons in sensory nerves in which sensory action potentials could be detected neither by surface nor by near-nerve needle electrodes after antidromic stimulation. Dyck et al found statistically significant and comparable improvement in the summed compound muscle action potentials at 6 weeks of treatment with IVIG or with plasma exchange, and they were correlated with improvement of motor function.[13]

In summary, although it is difficult to predict the outcome of CIDP, several factors have been identified that can help. A relapsing–remitting course, a younger age, and preservation of axons seem to indicate a good prognosis. Unfortunately a remitting course often becomes progressive after a few years, and axon loss increases gradually.

References

1. Gorson KC, Allam G, Ropper AH. Chronic inflammatory demyelinating polyneuropathy: clinical features and response to treatment in 67 consecutive patients with and without a monoclonal gammopathy. *Neurology* 1997; **48:** 321–328.

2. Bouchard C, Lacroix C, Planté V et al. Clinicopathologic findings and prognosis of chronic inflammatory demyelinating polyneuropathy. *Neurology* 1999; **52:** 498–503.

3. Nagamatsu M, Terao S, Misu K et al. Axonal and perikaryal involvement in chronic inflammatory demyelinating polyneuropathy. *J Neurol Neurosurg Psych* 1999; **66:** 727–733.

4. Said G, Hontebeyrie-Joskowicz M. Nerve lesions induced by macrophage activation. *Res Immunol* 1992; **143:** 589–599.

5. Asbury AK, Arnason B, Adams R. The inflammatory lesion in idiopathic polyneuritis: its role in pathogenesis. *Medicine* (Baltimore) 1969; **48:** 173–215.

6. Griffin JW, Li CY, Ho TW et al. Pathology of the motor-sensory axonal Guillain-Barré syndrome [see comments]. *Ann Neurol* 1996; **39:** 17–28.

7. Berciano J, Figols J, Garcia A et al. Fulminant Guillain-Barré syndrome with universal inexcitability of peripheral nerves: a clinicopathological study. *Muscle Nerve* 1997; **20:** 846–857.

8. Madrid R, Wiesniewski H. Axonal degeneration in demyelinating disorders. *J Neurocytol* 1977; **6:** 103–117.

9. Said G, Saida K, Saida T, Asbury AK. Axonal lesions in acute experimental demyelination: a sequential teased nerve fiber study. *Neurology* 1981; **31:** 421.

10. Van Doorn PA, Vermeulen M, Brand A et al. Intravenous immunoglobulin treatment in patients with chronic inflammatory demyelinating polyneuropathy. Clinical and laboratory characteristics associated with improvement. *Arch Neurol* 1991; **48:** 217–220.

11. Hahn AF, Bolton CF, Zochodne D, Feasby TE. Intravenous immunoglobulin treatment in chronic inflammatory demyelinating polyneuropathy. A double-blind, placebo-controlled, cross-over study. *Brain* 1996; **119:** 1067–1077.

12. Thompson N, Choudhary PP, Hughes RA, Quinlivan RM. A novel trial design to study the effect of intravenous immunoglobulin in chronic inflammatory demyelinating polyradiculoneuropathy. *J Neurol* 1996; **243**: 280–285.

13. Dyck PJ, Litchy WJ, Kratz KM et al. A plasma exchange versus immune globulin infusion trial in chronic inflammatory demyelinating polyradiculoneuropathy. *Ann Neurol* 1994; **36**: 838–845.

Inflammatory myopathies

Marinos C Dalakas

5

> DM: dermatomyositis; HIV: human immunodeficiency virus; HTLV-I: human T-cell lymphotrophic virus type I; IBM: inclusion body myositis; ICAM: intercellular cell adhesion molecule; IVIG: intravenous immunoglobulin; LEMS: Lambert–Eaton myasthenic syndrome; LFA: lymphocyte function-associated antigen; MAC: membranolytic attack complex; MHC: major histocompatibility complex; MRC: Medical Research Council; mRNA: messenger RNA; N-CAM: neural cell adhesion molecule; NIH: National Institutes of Health; PM: polymyositis; TGF: transforming growth factor

Introduction

The inflammatory myopathies are divided into three major and distinct subsets: polymyositis (PM), dermatomyositis (DM), and inclusion body myositis (IBM).[1–6] Although their cause is unknown, autoimmune mechanisms are implicated as supported by their association with other putative or definite autoimmune diseases or viruses, the evidence for a T-cell-mediated myocytotoxicity or complement-mediated microangiopathy, and the presence of various autoantibodies.[1-6] This is also true for IBM, in spite of the co-existence of various degenerative features in these patients' muscle biopsies.[7,8]

Clinical experience indicates that patients with PM and DM respond to prednisone in some degree and for varying periods.[9-11] In some patients the response may be dramatic, and if prudently used prednisone may have a long-lasting effect with minimal side-effects.[12] In other patients, however, the response is mild to moderate, and in still others, the steroid-induced side-effects are severe, necessitating the need for other immunosuppressive drugs. Azathioprine, methotrexate, cyclosporin, cyclophosphamide, and mycophendate are commonly used immunosuppressants which offer a mild or, at the very best, a modest benefit, but with considerable toxicity after long-term use. Plasmapheresis is ineffective.[13] IBM is almost always unresponsive to steroids or other immunosuppressants. The need for more effective therapies and the encouraging results from pilot or uncontrolled studies,[14-17] have prompted the need to examine the therapeutic efficacy of high-dose intravenous immunoglobulin (IVIG), an immunomodulating drug with prohibitive cost but minimal toxicity. This chapter summarizes the value of IVIG in inflammatory myopathies based on controlled studies performed at the National Institutes for Health (NIH) separately for PM, DM and IBM. The accessibility of muscle biopsy tissues before and after therapy has also offered the opportunity to study the mechanism of action of IVIG and provide information useful in understanding how IVIG works, not only in inflammatory myopathies but also in other autoimmune neurological disorders.

IVIG in dermatomyositis

Dermatomyositis affects the skeletal muscles, resulting in proximal muscle weakness, and also the skin, causing a characteristic violaceous rash on the face, chest, knees, back and the knuckles of the fingers.[1-6] Dilated or infarcted capillaries at the bases of the fingernails are frequently present. The muscle biopsy shows endomysial inflammation which is predominantly perivascular or in the interfascicular septa and around, rather than within, the fascicles. The earliest lesion that precedes inflammation or structural changes in the muscle fibers is the deposition of the complement C5b–9 membranolytic attack complex (MAC) on the intramuscular capillaries.[1-6,18,19] This is followed by necrosis and marked reduction in the number of capillaries per muscle fiber, especially in the perifascicular regions, resulting in ischemia and muscle fiber destruction that often resembles microinfarcts. Cytokines and adhesion molecules participate in the trafficking of sensitized lymphocytes and macrophages from the intramuscular blood vessels to the muscle fibers.[1-6] These molecules may be also responsible for the upregulation of the major histocompatibility complex (MHC) class I antigen expression on the muscle fibers, especially in the perifascicular regions, which are the areas most severely affected by the immunopathological process. Considering all the aforementioned immune mechanisms, if IVIG is effective in DM, one may expect to see not only clinical benefit but also improvement in the muscle cytoarchitecture, downregulation of cytokines or adhesion molecules, effect on the complement activation and MAC formation and improvement of the muscle microvasculature. Evidence that IVIG had an impressive effect in all these parameters is given below.

Results of a controlled study

To assess the effect of IVIG in patients with DM a double-blind, placebo-controlled study was conducted.[18] Patients incompletely responsive to various immunotherapeutic agents or those who had experienced significant side-effects from long-term steroid therapy were selected. A total of 15 patients (aged 18–55 years) with biopsy-proven, treatment-resistant dermatomyositis were randomly assigned to receive IVIG (a total of 2 g/kg daily) or placebo, every month for 3 months, with the option of crossing over to the alternative therapy for 3 more months after a wash-out period of 1 month. The patients continued to receive prednisone at a mean daily dose (25 mg) that remained unchanged for 3 months before and after therapy. Clinical response was gauged by assessing changes in:

(a) muscle strength, using a modified MRC scale, a well-validated scale in the treatment of neuromuscular disorders;
(b) scores of neuromuscular symptoms that provide a picture of the daily living activities;
(c) the rash, using photography under the same lighting conditions.

Details of the methodology and scales were previously reported.[18] Further, a histological and immunopathological improvement was sought on the basis of quantitative histochemistry and immunopathology performed in repeated muscle biopsies.

Of the 15 patients, eight were assigned to IVIG and seven to placebo. Their scores at randomization and the mean disease duration in years were similar in both groups (*Table 5.1*).[18] The patients randomized to IVIG had a significant improvement in the scores of muscle strength, from a mean of 76.6 ± 5.7

to 84.6 ± 4.6, and in the neuromuscular symptoms scores, from a mean of 44 ± 8.2 to 51.4 ± 6. In contrast, the seven patients assigned to placebo did not change and their scores remained the same, from 78.6 ± 6.3 to 78.6 ± 8.2 and from 45.9 ± 9.0 to 45.7 ± 11.3, respectively (*Table 5.1*). The difference in scores between baseline and end of treatment among IVIG and placebo-treated patients was significant ($P < 0.018$ for the muscle strength and $P < 0.035$ for the neuromuscular symptoms). With crossovers, a total of 12 patients received IVIG; of those, nine with severe disabilities had a major improvement (defined as more than 5 grades increase in the MRC scores) reaching nearly normal function, two had mild improvement and one had no change (*Table 5.2*). The mean muscle strength scores in these nine patients increased from 74.5 ± 4.9 to 84.7 ± 4.5. Their neuromuscular symptoms also improved significantly, from 38.6 ± 5.9 to 51 ± 8.0.[19] The statistically significant improvements in muscle strength, expressed as MRC and neuromuscular symptoms scores, were functionally impressive for individual patients, some of whom were wheelchair-bound before therapy and walked independently or regained full strength after 3 months of IVIG. Of 11 placebo-treated patients, none had major improvement, three had mild improvement, three had no change in their condition, and five worsened (*Table 5.2*).

The improvement became noticeable about 15 days after the first IVIG infusion and it was clear and definitive after the second infusion. Only two of the responders reached their peak after the second infusion; the rest peaked between the second and third infusions. Eight patients had marked improvement of the active violaceous rash, or the chronic scaly eruptions on their knuckles, which often preceded or coincided with the improvement of muscle strength. Serum creatine kinase levels, elevated up to 10-fold in seven of the IVIG-treated patients, fell by 50% after the first infusion and decreased further or normalized by the second infusion. Creatine kinase levels remained elevated, were unchanged, or increased during placebo, and returned to baseline 6–10 weeks after the IVIG-treated patients crossed over to placebo or the IVIG infusions were stopped. Overall, the patients who noted major improvement felt that IVIG had a serious impact on their daily activities, without troublesome adverse effects.

In subsequent open-labeled infusions, the benefit of IVIG was also documented in more than 15 patients treated by the author's group or under our supervision in several institutions. The improvement was also documented in one of the open-label-treated patients using quantitative muscle strength testing—the maximal voluntary isometric contractions method—which measures changes in muscle strength in newtons.[20] In this patient, the scores improved from 202 N

Table 5.1
Response to IVIG in a placebo-controlled study of patients with dermatomyositis. Values are mean manual muscle strength (MRC) scores and mean neuromuscular symptom (NS) scores.

Therapy	Mean duration of disease (years)	Pretreatment		After treatment*	
		MRC	NS	MRC	NS
IVIG (n = 8)	3.9	76.6 ± 5.7	44.1 ± 8.2	84.6 ± 4.6†	51.4 ± 6.0‡
Placebo (n = 7)	3.8	78.6 ± 6.3	45.9 ± 9.0	78.6 ± 8.2	45.7 ± 11.3

*Response to IVIG or placebo was measured after 3 months of treatment and before crossover to the alternative therapy, the effect of which is shown in Fig. 5.1 (see text for details).
†P = 0.018 (Wilcoxon) for comparison with placebo value.
‡P = 0.035 (Wilcoxon) for comparison with placebo value.

Table 5.2
Response to IVIG in a placebo-controlled study of patients with dermatomyositis, including a crossover phase.

Response	Placebo (n = 11)	IVIG (n = 12)
Major improvement*	0	9
Mild improvement†	3	2
No change	3	1
Deterioration	5	0

*Defined as a more than 5-grade increase in both the total MRC score and the total neuromuscular symptom score.
†Defined as an increase of 2–5 grades in the total MRC score and the total neuromuscular symptom score.

at baseline to 358 N after the third infusion. She used a cane to walk before therapy but became able to exercise on parallel bars after two IVIG infusions.[19]

Role of IVIG in maintaining response

The improvement in strength is usually short-lived, not lasting more than 4–8 weeks. Most of the original patients from this study continue to receive IVIG and respond to a variable degree. Some patients need IVIG less frequently and continue to maintain their improvement in conjunction with low-dose steroids; two patients who were wheelchair-bound prior to therapy and received IVIG for 2 years have maintained normal strength without any drugs for 3–5 years; others need IVIG every 3–4 weeks to maintain excellent response; and some others continue to improve on 4–6 week regimens but the improvement is not as impressive as initially, presumably because of further progression of the disease or a diminished response to IVIG therapy. In several patients it was possible to lower the prednisone dose and keep it at a low maintenance level. It is the author's experience that low-dose prednisone is helpful and appears to enhance the benefit of IVIG. It was also noted that some patients who had become unresponsive to steroids responded again to prednisone after a few infusions with IVIG. The phenomenon of restoring responsiveness to steroids is an interesting one and needs to be further studied, not only in DM but also in chronic inflammatory demyelinating polyneuropathy where it has been also noted (author's unpublished observations).

How IVIG exerts its action: studies on repeated muscle biopsies and on post-IVIG sera

In patients who showed major improvement, repeat open muscle biopsies on the biceps muscle opposite the one used for the pretreatment biopsy were performed 15 days after the last IVIG infusion. Before the code was broken, the pretreatment biopsies were processed for muscle enzyme histochemistry and immunocytochemistry in an immunoperoxidase technique, using antibodies against MHC-I, ICAM-I, Leu-19 (to assess the regenerating muscle fibers) and various lymphocyte subsets[15] and TGFβ protein and mRNA. Further, the capillaries were visualized by immunofluorescence and immunoperoxidase staining, using the lectin *Ulex europaeus*, which stains the capillary endothelial cells.[18,19] In five randomly selected perifascicular regions at a low, original (×40) magnification, each region corresponding to a large 6.4×10^4 μm² surface area, the number of capillaries and their diameter were noted, as well as the number of muscle fibers and their diameter, and the ratio of muscle fiber to capillaries was calculated (*Table 5.3* and *Fig. 5.1*). The biopsy measurements following treatment were compared not only with the pretreatment biopsies but also with five biopsies from patients with limb-girdle dystrophies who served as disease controls.

A marked improvement in muscle histology was noted in the repeated biopsies compared with the pre-IVIG biopsies. As shown in *Table 5.3*, the mean number of

Table 5.3
Effect of IVIG on histological characteristics in the muscles of patients with dermatomyositis.

	Pretreatment (n = 5)	After treatment (n = 5)
Muscle fibers*	34.2 ± 2	24.8 ± 8
Muscle fiber diameter (μm)	54 ± 11	71 ± 15†
Capillaries*	13.5 ± 3	18.2 ± 4.8 (normal 19.7 ± 6.7)
Capillary diameter (μm)	11.0 ± 2.8	7.4 ± 2‡ (normal 6.5 ± 0.01)
Muscle fiber : capillaries	3.4	1.54 (normal 1.2)

*Mean number of muscle fibers or capillaries in five randomly selected perifascicular regions at a low, original ×40 magnification, each region corresponding to a 6.4×10^4 μm² surface area (see text for details).
†P = 0.04 (ANOVA) for comparison with pretreatment value.
‡P = 0.01 (ANOVA) for comparison with pretreatment value.

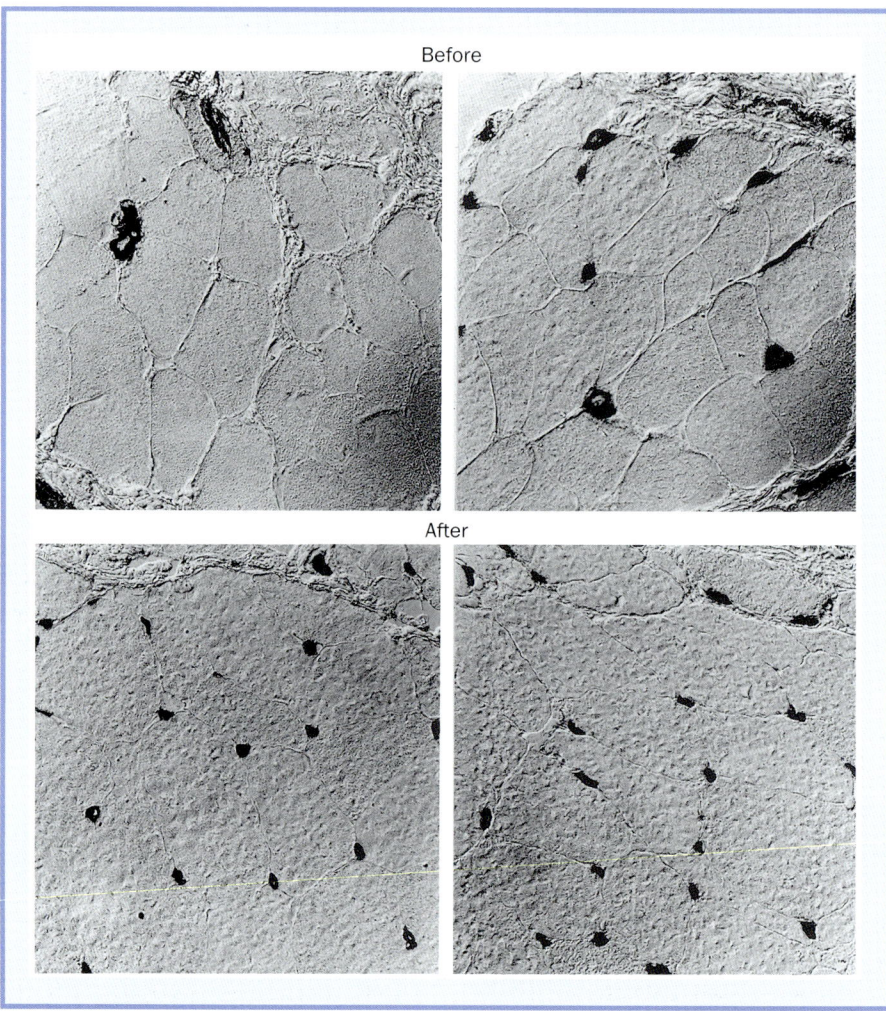

Figure 5.1
Cross-section of representative muscle areas before therapy (top panels) and after therapy (lower panels) stained for Ulex europaeus which identifies the endothelial cells (see quantification of capillaries in Table 5.3). An increase in the number of capillaries and reduction in fiber diameter is shown after therapy (lower panels). The same magnification is used for both.

muscle fibers counted in the five regions decreased as a result of an increase in the muscle fiber diameter, from a mean of 54.0 ± 11 μm to 71.0 ± 15 μm ($P < 0.04$). The mean number of capillaries increased and their mean diameter decreased from 11.0 ± 3 μm to 7.4 ± 2 μm (normal, 6.5 ± 0.1 μm) ($P < 0.01$) (*Table 5.3*). The mean ratio of muscle fibers to capillaries also decreased from 3.4 to 1.5 (normal 1.2) and normalized in three patients (*Table 5.3*).

Among the main immunological markers on the repeated biopsy was the downregulation of the MHC-I molecule which was markedly expressed in the pretreatment biopsy in the perifascicular regions (*Fig. 5.2*). In addition, the ICAM-I expression on the surface of some muscle fibers and on the blood vessels was suppressed after IVIG therapy.[18] Because ICAM-I, the ligand for LFA-I, was overexpressed on the endothelial cells before therapy, the IVIG-induced downregulation of ICAM-I probably had an effect on the exit of activated T cells from the capillaries towards the muscle fibers, and might have been responsible for the reduction of inflammatory cells noted in the repeated biopsies. Another effect of IVIG was on TGFβ expression. TGFβ is a pleotropic cytokine which, when in excess, induces chronic inflammation and fibrosis. In the tissues of DM patients, TGFβ is upregulated both at the protein and the mRNA level.[20]

After IVIG, the repeated muscle biopsies revealed an impressive downregulation of TGFβ and the TGFβ mRNA. Interestingly, this effect was not observed in five repeated muscle biopsies from patients with inclusion body myositis who did not respond to IVIG, as discussed below.[20]

The most remarkable improvement in reference to the immunopathogenetic mechanism of DM was the IVIG-induced interception of the formation and intramuscular deposition of the membranolytic attack complex, the lytic component of the complement pathway. In the repeat muscle biopsies, the C3bNEO (neoantigen) which is immune-complex specific, and the MAC could not be detected in the endomysial capillaries.[21–23] Further, in an assay system of in vitro sensitized erythrocytes the consumption of C3 uptake by the patients' sera was suppressed after IVIG, compared with the pretreatment sera.[22] As discussed in the mechanism of action of IVIG,[24,25] IVIG inhibited the incorporation of C3 into the C5 convertase assembly, prevented the formation of C3bNEO (see *Fig. 5.3*)[24] and intercepted the formation and deposition of MAC on the endomysial capillaries. Consequently, IVIG allowed neovascularization and the reversal of the ischemic process, as demonstrated by the normalization of the capillaries and the muscle fiber diameter in the repeat muscle biopsies (see *Figs 5.1* and *5.2*).

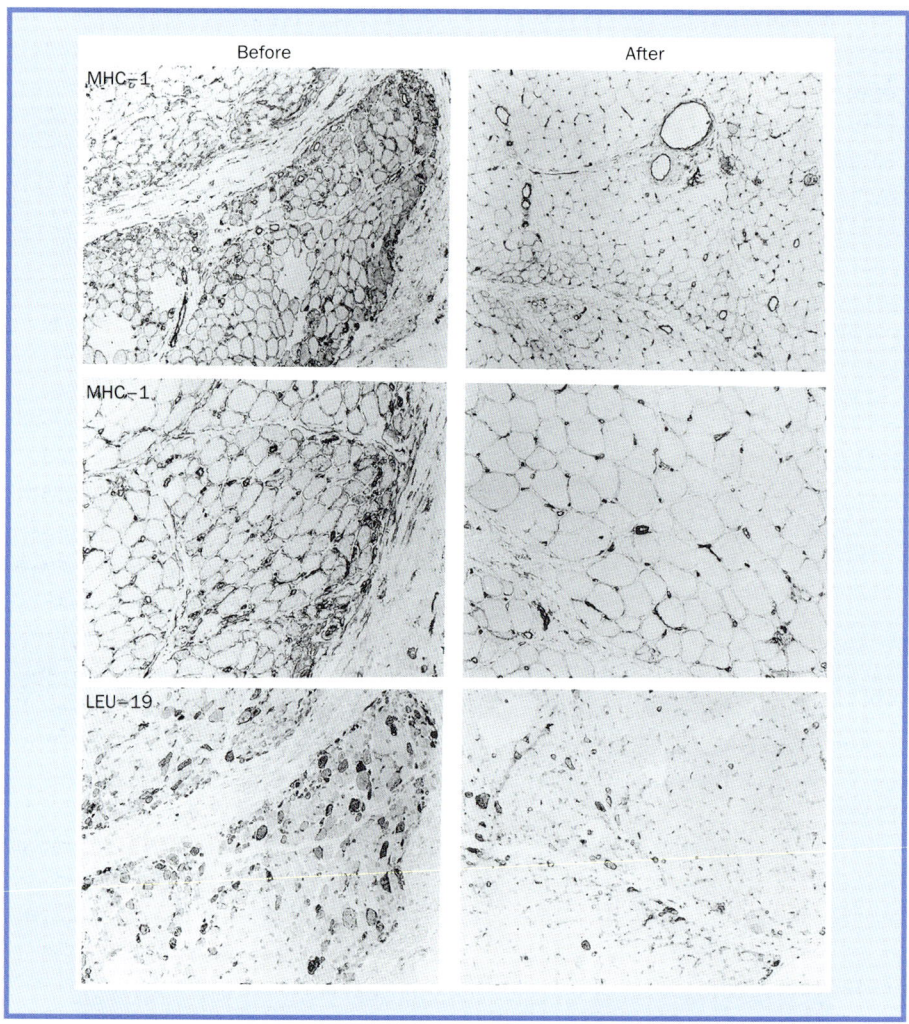

Figure 5.2
Cross-section of muscle biopsies stained for MHC-I (top and middle figure) and for Leu-19 (low figure) before (left) and after IVIG therapy (right) shows the marked suppression of MHC-I expression and the downregulation of Leu-19-positive fibers. The increase in the diameter of the muscle fibers especially in the periphery is prominent after therapy. The perivascular inflammatory responses seen before, as MHC-positive cells, improved after therapy. Two MHC-I figures are shown (top and middle) at different magnifications.

The effect of IVIG to intercept the formation and deposition of MAC in target tissues may be also relevant to other IVIG-responsive diseases in which tissue damage is mediated by complement activation and MAC deposition. For example, MAC deposition mediates the destruction not only of the capillaries in DM but also of the myelin sheath in Guillain–Barré syndrome and the acetylcholine receptors in myasthenia gravis.

IVIG in inclusion body myositis

Inclusion body myositis is the most common acquired inflammatory myopathy in patients over the age of 50 years.[1–8] The condition presents with selective atrophy of the forearm flexor muscles, frequent falls, atrophy of the quadriceps muscles, and dysphagia. The histological hallmarks of IBM are:

(a) basophilic granular inclusions distributed around the edge of slit-like vacuoles (rimmed vacuoles);
(b) angulated or round fibers, often in small groups;
(c) eosinophilic cytoplasmic inclusions;
(d) prominent endomysial inflammation in a pattern identical to that seen in PM;
(e) Congo red or crystal violet positive staining of amyloid deposits next to the vacuoles.

Controlled trials

In an open pilot trial, IVIG seemed to be helpful in some patients with IBM because the strength improved in some muscle groups after treatment.[17] Although the improvement was not dramatic, it made a difference to the patients' life styles. Another uncontrolled series of patients collected from three institutions showed no benefit from IVIG.[26] Subsequently, a controlled, double-blind study involving 19 patients with IBM was conducted at the NIH.[27] Efficacy was assessed by quantitative muscle strength testing and quantification of swallowing function, which is so commonly affected in IBM patients. The study, a 3-month, randomized, crossover trial, was designed similarly to the one described earlier for DM. No statistically significant differences were noted in the strength of the limb muscles between placebo and IVIG (*Fig. 5.3*). Whether the small sample size might have been a factor is unknown. However, regional significant differences were observed in the IVIG-randomized patients, especially in the muscles of swallowing measured objectively by the ultrasound technique.[27] As shown in *Table 5.4*, the duration of swallow was statistically significant in the IVIG-randomized patients compared with placebo. The nonsignificant effect in the limb muscles, compared with the swallowing muscles, might have been due to the more precise, objective and reproducible measurement of the

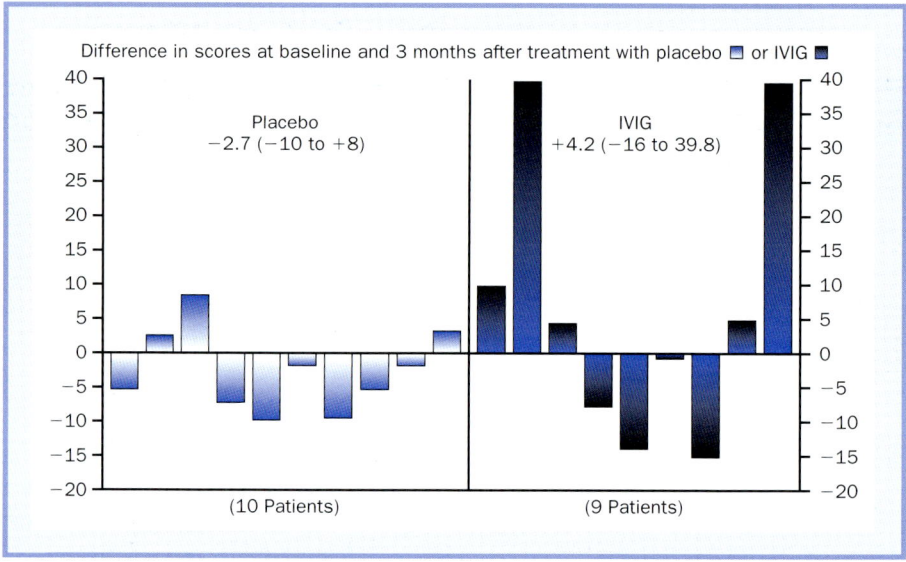

Figure 5.3
Differences in MRC scores at baseline and 3 months after treatment. Open bars represent individual patients initially randomized to placebo and closed bars those randomized to IVIG. The placebo-randomized patients lost a mean of 2.7 MRC points and the IVIG-randomized patients gained overall 4.2 points, but the difference between the two groups was not significant. Even though, as a group, the IVIG-treated patients did not differ significantly from the placebo, in six patients (1, 2, 9 in the figure and three others who improved when they crossed over to IVIG after placebo) the improvement was functionally important for their daily activities.

swallowing function. Because the test-to-test variability with the ultrasound technique that measures the duration of swallowing in seconds is minimal, this technique allows us to capture even minor improvements.

Although in the limb muscles the study did not overall establish efficacy of IVIG, six of 19 IBM patients (28%) showed a mild improvement in muscle strength which was functionally important for their daily activities (*Fig. 5.3*). Because IBM patients do not respond to therapies and the disease is incapacitating, even a minor improvement may have a positive impact for some of the patients' functions. On this basis a larger study was conducted, combining this time IVIG with prednisone. This was a double-blind, placebo-controlled study involving 37 patients, 19 of whom were randomized to IVIG plus high-dose steroids and 18 to

Table 5.4
Mean duration (seconds) of ultrasound swallows at baseline, 3 months, and end of crossover of 19 patients with IBM treated with placebos or IVIG.

	Type of swallow	Baseline	3 months	Crossover
			Placebo	**IVIG**
Patients randomized to placebo (n = 10)*	D1	2.33	1.83	1.91
	D2	2.15	1.75	1.88
	D3	1.84**	2.84**	1.83**
	W1	1.59**	2.25**	1.86**
	W2	2.49	1.96	2.00
	W3	1.59**	2.07**	2.44*
			IVIG	**Placebo**
Patients randomized to IVIG (n = 9)*	D1	3.00**	1.62**	1.47
	D2	3.37**	2.02**	2.31
	D3	2.35	2.74**	1.85**
	W1	1.82	1.86	1.47
	W2	1.73**	1.24**	1.54
	W3	1.98**	1.49**	1.48

*P = 0.05.
**P = 0.05.

placebo plus high-dose steroids.[28,29] The changes in muscle strength were assessed with quantitative muscle strength testing and the MRC scale. After 3 months of treatment, there was no clear benefit in any of the two groups. Minor gains in strength were noted in the IVIG-randomized patients but were not significant. Subjective improvements were noted in 10 of the 19 patients randomized to IVIG compared with 1 of 18 randomized to placebo. The repeated muscle biopsies showed a reduction in the T cell count in both groups, probably related to steroids. No changes in the muscle cytoarchitecture, vacuoles, amyloid deposits or adhesion molecules (N-CAM) were noted. The TGFβ in the muscle remained unchanged both at the protein and the mRNA level.[20] This is in contrast to the TGFβ in DM patients, which was downregulated and correlated with clinical improvement as discussed earlier. This second study also failed to show efficacy of IVIG.

In spite of these two negative trials, it is the author's clinical impression that a few patients may show transient signs of improvement which are minor and difficult to capture with the methods used but can be clinically significant for the patients' activities and life styles, at least temporarily. Whether such a mild improvement in a small number of IBM patients justifies a 2–3 month trial with IVIG remains a matter of clinical judgment, and should be viewed on a case-by-case basis. The noted statistical improvement in the swallowing muscles (*Table 5.4*) may be a factor for considering IVIG in selected patients with significant dysphagia. Safety, age, economics, and the reminder that nothing else (including steroids) offers even minor clinical improvement to IBM patients should be also taken into account.

IVIG in polymyositis

In PM and IBM, there is evidence not of microangiopathy and muscle ischemia, as in DM, but of an antigen-directed cytotoxicity mediated by cytotoxic T cells.[1–8] This conclusion is supported by the presence of CD8+ T cells, which along with macrophages, initially surround healthy, nonnecrotic muscle fibers and eventually invade and destroy. The muscle fibers, either next to or remote from the areas of inflammation, strongly express the MHC class I antigen, which is absent from the sarcolemma of normal muscle fibers.[2–4] Because cytotoxic T cells recognize antigenic targets in association with MHC-I antigen, the primary immunopathological mechanism in PM and IBM is T-cell-mediated and MHC-I antigen restricted. The immunopathology is almost identical in both PM and IBM even if the latter does not respond to immunotherapies.

In uncontrolled studies, IVIG has been shown to be effective in PM.[14,15] However, controlled studies using quantitative muscle strength testing and documentation of the disease with muscle biopsies prior to therapy have not yet been completed. Such a controlled clinical trial in PM began at the NIH more than 7 years ago, but it has not yet been completed because most patients referred as having PM resistant to therapy turn out to have IBM or something else. Although from the enrolled patients the clinical impression is that IVIG appears to be helpful in carefully selected PM patients, the study code is not yet broken and the results in the few patients we treated have not been analyzed.

IVIG in retroviral-associated polymyositis

Polymyositis and IBM can be seen in association with HIV and HTLV-I infection.[30–32] In these conditions, the virus does not infect the muscle but it triggers a T-cell-mediated inflammatory response that is immunopathologically identical to the one described in retroviral-negative PM.[30–32]

In three patients treated in a controlled crossover trial, only minimal changes in the patient's strength were noted after IVIG, compared with placebo. Although the series is small, these results do not support the efficacy of IVIG.

References

1. Dalakas MC. Polymyositis, dermatomyositis, and inclusion-body myositis. *New Engl J Med* 1991; **325:** 1487–1498.

2. Engel AG, Hohlfeld R, Banker BQ. The polymyositis and dermatomyositis syndrome. In: Engel AG, Franzini-Armstrong C, eds. *Myology*. New York: McGraw-Hill, 1994, 1335–1383.

3. Karpati G, Carpenter S. Pathology of the inflammatory myopathies. In: Mastaglia FL, ed. *Baillière's Clinical Neurology*. London: WB Saunders, 1993, 527–556.

4. Dalakas MC. Immunopathogenesis of inflammatory myopathies. *Ann Neurol* 1995; **37:** 74–86.

5. Dalakas MC. Immunopathogenesis of inflammatory myopathies. In: Antel JP, Birnbaum G, Hartung HP, eds. *Clinical Neuroimmunology*. Cambridge: Blackwell Science, 1998, 374–384.

6. Sivakumar K, Dalakas MC. Inclusion body myositis and myopathies. *Curr Opin Neurol* 1997; **10:** 413–420.

7. Koffman BM, Sivakumar K, Simonis T et al. HLA allele distribution distinguishes sporadic inclusion body myositis from hereditary inclusion body myopathies. *J Neuroimmunol* 1998; **84:** 139–142.

8. Koffman BM, Rugiero M, Dalakas MC. Autoimmune diseases and autoantibodies associated with sporadic inclusion body myositis. *Muscle Nerve* 1998; **21:** 115–117.

9. Dalakas MC. How to diagnose and treat the inflammatory myopathies. *Semin Neurol* 1994; **14:** 137–45.

10. Dalakas MC. The treatment of polymyositis, dermatomyositis and inclusion body myositis. In: Johnson RT, Griffin JW, eds. *Current Therapy in Neurology*. St Louis: Mosby/Year Book, 1996, 407–412.

11. Dalakas MC. Polymyositis, dermatomyositis and inclusion body myositis. In: Kassirer JP, Greene HL, eds. *Current Therapy in Adult Medicine*. St Louis: Mosby/Year Book, 1997, 1434–1439.

12. Dalakas, MC. Treatment of polymyositis and dermatomyositis. *Curr Opin Rheumatol* 1989; **1:** 443–449.

13. Miller FW, Leitman SF, Cronin ME et al. Controlled trial of plasma exchange and leukopheresis in polymyositis and dermatomyositis. *New Engl J Med* 1992; **326:** 1380–1384.

14. Cherin P, Herson S, Wechsler B et al. Efficacy of intravenous immunoglobulin therapy in chronic refractory polymyositis and dermatomyositis. An open study with 20 adult patients. *Am J Med* 1991; **91:** 162–168.

15. Lang B, Laxer RM, Murphy G et al. Treatment of dermatomyositis with intravenous immunoglobulin. *Am J Med* 1991; **91:** 169–172.

16. Jan S, Beretta S, Moggio M et al. High-dose intravenous human immunoglobulin in polymyositis resistant to treatment. *J Neurol Neurosurg Psych* 1992; **55:** 60–64.

17. Soueidan SA, Dalakas MC. Treatment of inclusion-body myositis with high-dose

intravenous immunoglobulin. *Neurology* 1993; **43**: 876–879.

18. Dalakas MC, Illa I, Dambrosia JM et al. A controlled trial of high-dose intravenous immunoglobulin infusions as treatment for dermatomyositis. *New Engl J Med* 1993; **329**: 1993–2000.

19. Dalakas MC. Intravenous immune globulin for dermatomyositis. *New Engl J Med* 1994; **330**: 1392–1393.

20. Amemiya K, Semino-Mora C, Granger RP, Dalakas MC. Down regulation of TGF-b_1, mRNA and protein in the muscle of patients with inflammatory myopathy after treatment with high-dose intravenous immunoglobulin. *Clin Immunol* 2000; **94**: 99–104.

21. Dalakas MC. Experience with IVIg in the treatment of inflammatory myopathies. In: Kazatchkine L, Morel M, eds. *Intravenous Immunoglobulin Research and Therapy*. New York: Parthenon, 1996, 275–284.

22. Basta M, Dalakas MC. High-dose intravenous immunoglobulin exerts its beneficial effect in patients with dermatomyositis by blocking endomysial deposition of activated complement fragments. *J Clin Invest* 1994; **94**: 1729–1735.

23. Dalakas MC. Clinical relevance of IVIg in the modulation of the complement-mediated tissue damage: implications in dermatomyositis, Guillain–Barré syndrome and myasthenia gravis. In: Kazatchkine L, Morel M, eds. *Intravenous Immunoglobulin Research and Therapy*. New York: Parthenon, 1996, 89–93.

24. Dalakas MC. Mechanism of action of intravenous immunoglobulin and therapeutic considerations in the treatment of autoimmune neurologic diseases. *Neurology* 1998; **51 (suppl 5)**: S2–S8.

25. Dalakas MC. Intravenous immunoglobulin in the treatment of autoimmune neuromuscular diseases: present status and practical therapeutic guidelines. *Muscle Nerve* 1999; **22**: 1479–1497.

26. Amato AA, Barohn RJ, Jackson CE et al. Inclusion body myositis: treatment with intravenous immunoglobulin. *Neurology* 1993; **43**: 876–879.

27. Dalakas MC, Sonies B, Dambrosia J et al. Treatment of inclusion body, myositis with IVIg: a double-blind, placebo-control study. *Neurology* 1997; **48**: 712–716.

28. Dalakas MC, Sonies B, Koffman B et al. High-dose intravenous immunoglobulin (IVIg) combined with prednisone in the treatment of patients with inclusion-body myositis (IBM): a double blind, randomised controlled trial. *Neurology* 1997; **48**: 332.

29. Dalakas MC. Controlled studies with high-dose intravenous immunoglobulin in the treatment of dermatomyositis, inclusion body myositis and polymyositis. *Neurology* 1998; **51(suppl 5)**: 537–545.

30. Dalakas MC, Pezeshkpour GH, Gravell M, Sever JL. Polymyositis in patients with AIDS. *JAMA* 1986; **256**: 2381–2383.

31. Dalakas MC, Pezeshkpour GH. Neuromuscular diseases associated with human immunodeficiency virus infection. *Ann Neurol* 1988; **23(S)**: 38–48.

32. Cupler EJ, Leon-Monzon M, Miller J et al. Inclusion body myositis in HIV-1 and HTLV-1 infected patients. *Brain* 1996; **119**: 1887–1893.

Guillain–Barré syndrome

David R Cornblath

6

> AIDP: acute inflammatory demyelinating polyneuropathy; AMAN: acute motor axonal neuropathy; AMSAN: acute motor sensory axonal neuropathy; GBS: Guillain–Barré syndrome; IVIG: intravenous immunoglobulin; PE: plasma exchange

Introduction

The 1990s have seen an explosion in knowledge concerning the Guillain–Barré syndrome (GBS). This has resulted from concerted efforts by many groups around the world to improve the understanding and treatment of this syndrome.

GBS initially was defined by clinical and spinal fluid features.[1,2] Following the swine flu incident,[3] the US National Institute of Neurological Disorders and Stroke set up a task force to define the syndrome explicitly for epidemiological purposes.[4] The task force defined the cardinal clinical features, including progressive motor weakness of more than one limb, hyporeflexia or areflexia, with maximum deficit reached within 4 weeks. In addition, spinal fluid criteria were proposed which carried forth the original observations by Guillain, Barré, and Strohl[2] of an albuminocytologic dissociation in the spinal fluid. Other similar syndromes must be excluded to leave the syndromic diagnosis of GBS. At the time these criteria were written, it was implied that cases of GBS were associated with peripheral nerve demyelination as detected by electrophysiology or pathology and inflammation as detected by nerve biopsy or autopsy. This notion of an acute inflammatory demyelinating polyneuropathy (AIDP), a term still used today as synonymous with GBS, came from careful electrophysiological[5,6] and pathological[7-9] studies. As a result of these and experimental studies (see below), the notion was put forward that GBS was an immune-mediated, inflammatory, demyelinating, peripheral nerve disorder caused by invading lymphocytes and recruited macrophages.[7] These notions, which have stood the test of time, represent only part of the complete syndrome, however.

In 1986, Feasby et al proposed that there was an acute fulminant form of GBS in which the primary attack was on the axon and not the myelin as in the AIDP form.[10] Initially, many were skeptical of this notion as the data presented could have been consistent with a severe, massive attack on the myelin sheath with secondary axon loss from the 'bystander effect'. The electrophysiologic features in this syndrome were characterized by absent or severely reduced motor and sensory evoked amplitudes, but these could be seen with either severe terminal demyelination or severe axon loss, either primary or secondary. The autopsy studies were performed late in the illness, and therefore it might have been that an acute attack on the myelin sheath could no longer be detected pathologically. Thus, the place of an axonal form of GBS remained controversial.

Studies in China by a joint Chinese–American group have significantly expanded our understanding of GBS.[11–21] In northern China, a disorder clinically similar to classical GBS or AIDP occurs, but in epidemics peaking during the summer months, and predominantly involving children and young adults.[11] Electrodiagnostic studies in this group suggest dysfunction of the motor axon primarily, in that motor conduction studies are characterized by low evoked amplitudes without features of demyelination. Sensory conduction studies are normal.[11] Neuropathological studies in this group of clinically and electrodiagnostically defined patients have convincingly shown an excellent correlation of the pathological and physiological studies.[12,14,16] These acute motor axonal neuropathy (AMAN) cases show isolated axonal dysfunction with only rare evidence of demyelination or inflammation.

Additional studies from China have shown that the initial notions put forward by Feasby et al were correct and that another form of GBS is an attack on the axons of both motor and sensory fibers, an acute motor sensory axonal neuropathy (AMSAN).[14,16,22]

Described in 1956, the Fisher syndrome, a clinical triad of ataxia, areflexia, and ophthalmoplegia, has been considered part of GBS.[23] The initial reasoning behind this was the similarities in clinical and spinal fluid features and the fact that some typical GBS patients had features seen in the Fisher syndrome.

A number of other clinical syndromes of more limited scope have also been described and included within GBS.[24]

Electrophysiology

Electrophysiological studies have played a key role in advancing our understanding of the disease. First, electrodiagnostic studies have clearly shown the heterogeneity of GBS.[11,25–29] In the AIDP form, nerve conductions are characterized by evidence of peripheral nerve demyelination, long recognized by abnormalities of the speed of conduction along nerve fibers, prolonged distal or F wave latencies and reduced conduction velocities, or evidence of conduction failure along the nerve resulting in partial motor conduction block. These features form the basis of identifying cases of AIDP among those with clinically defined GBS. In Australia, North America, and Europe, these electrodiagnostic features identify the majority of patients with clinically defined GBS as having AIDP.[26]

Conversely, the AMAN form of the disorder is characterized by nerve conduction studies suggesting axon loss or axon dysfunction purely along motor fibers.[11,25,29] Distal motor evoked amplitudes are moderately to severely reduced. The motor conduction parameters are normal unless the motor evoked amplitudes are severely reduced, and there is a concomitant conduction failure of the fast conducting nerve fibers. Thus, in the majority of cases, conduction velocity, distal and F wave latencies are normal. Sensory conduction studies are normal.

In the AMSAN form, both motor and sensory conduction studies are characterized by axonal loss or axonal dysfunction.[10]

In the Fisher syndrome, the most widely found abnormality is a gradual disappearance of sensory action potentials with their gradual reappearance with clinical improvement.[30] Because demyelination is so difficult to detect in sensory fibers, at face value it may be uncertain as to whether this is dysfunction of the myelin or the axon, but the rapid reappearance of sensory action potentials suggest that this is demyelination and not axon loss. If it were the latter, the return of sensory action potentials would take considerable time, as the nerves would have to regenerate.

A point of controversy has been the identification of peripheral nerve demyelination in the Guillain–Barré syndrome. Multiple schemes to identify peripheral nerve demyelination have been put forward, and there remains no universal consensus. In an effort to reconcile these differences, Alam et al compared several of these schema, finding that the four most commonly used provided similar results in identifying patients with peripheral nerve demyelination during the height of their illness.[31]

Lastly, multiple studies have shown the prognostic value of electrodiagnostic studies.[26,32,33] In most, the size of the distal evoked amplitude either combined from multiple muscles or in a single nerve, has been the best correlate of prognosis. Low motor evoked amplitudes define a group of patients with a protracted disease and a poor outcome.

Immunology

That GBS is an immunopathologically mediated disorder is unquestionable.[34–36] The initial observations suggesting this included the parallels to the experimental model, experimental allergic neuritis,[37,38] reports of improvement with immunotherapies,[39–42] and pathological studies showing inflammatory cells.[7,9] More recent immunopathological studies have suggested that in the AIDP form of GBS, there is an immunopathological attack on the Schwann cell plasmalemma resulting in demyelination.[43] Conversely, in the AMAN and AMSAN forms of GBS, immunopathological studies have suggested an immunopathological attack on axolemma[44] causing nodal dysfunction with the suggestion that the immunoepitope resides on the axonal membrane which is exposed at the node.[20,21]

Current thinking on the pathogenesis of GBS involves the process of molecular mimicry as the sequence of immunopathological events.[34–36,45] In the AIDP form, following an exciting infection, a host response is raised to the inciting events which cross-reacts with myelin. This cross-reactive response in the setting of the appropriate host results in peripheral nerve demyelination with immunoglobulin deposition and complement activation on the Schwann cell plasmalemma. In the AMAN form of the disorder, a similar inciting event, in many cases infection associated with *Campylobacter jejuni* enteritis, results in a cross-reactive response to axonal membrane components, the deposition of immunoglobulin, and then binding and activation of complement resulting in nodal dysfunction. In severe cases, macrophages may enter the nerve fiber under the myelin sheath, displacing or destroying the axon.

Considerable work continues on the role of gangliosides and antiganglioside antibodies in the pathogenesis of GBS. The current most convincing data involve the Fisher syndrome in which upwards of 90% of patients have anti-GQ1b antibodies in serum.[46–49] Further studies have shown that the antibody can be shown to bind to cranial motor nerves providing clinical pathologic correlation.[50]

Therapy

Plasma exchange

Beginning in the late 1970s and early 1980s, anecdotal reports began to appear that plasma exchange (PE) accelerated recovery in patients with GBS. Shortly thereafter, two large controlled clinical trials from North America[39] and France[40] convincingly proved that plasma exchange improves the outcome in patients with severe GBS, that is, those unable to walk independently, bed-bound, or on a ventilator. In the North American study, 245 patients were randomly assigned to PE, delivered as a total of 200–250 ml of plasma per kilogram, or to no therapy. A blinded assessor rated the patients at prescribed intervals. Patients receiving PE improved quicker, in particular in time to ambulation (53 days in the PE-treated group versus 85 days in the no-treatment group) and in time on a ventilator (24 days and 48 days, respectively). The French study included a similar number of patients, 220, randomly assigned to plasma exchange or sham exchange. Similar results were found. While a number of adverse events due to plasma exchange were noted, mortality rates in the two groups were similar in both studies.

Intravenous immunoglobulin therapy

Based on case reports,[51] interest began to develop in testing whether intravenous immunoglobulin (IVIG) therapy was also useful in treatment of Guillain–Barré syndrome. Since PE had previously been shown to be effective, a placebo-controlled clinical trial was not ethically possible. In the first randomized controlled study of IVIG in GBS, the Dutch Study Group compared IVIG 400 mg/kg per day for 5 days and PE 200–250 mg/kg plasma over 4–5 days.[41] In this study, IVIG was found to be at least equivalent to PE in improving patients.

Because of lingering concerns that the treatments indeed may not be equivalent, and because of reports of relapse following IVIG treatment,[52,53] a randomized controlled clinical trial was undertaken comparing IVIG, PE, or PE followed by a course of IVIG.[42] Of the 379 equally randomized subjects, there were no statistically significant differences among the three groups in the outcome measures: mean change in disability grade 4 weeks after therapy, number of patients ventilated after randomization, mean days to stop artificial respiration, median days to walking unaided, median days to hospital discharge, or median days to return to work. Thus, with these two studies,[41,42] IVIG was considered a standard of care in the treatment of severe GBS.

Three important features of these therapeutic studies should be noted. First, only patients who had severe GBS (unable to walk independently, bed-bound, or ventilator-dependent) were entered. Patients able to walk independently were not randomized. Thus, a quandary remained as to how to treat the patient with 'mild' GBS.

The French have provided evidence to suggest that indeed plasma exchange is valuable in these 'mild' patients.[54] In a study of 556 GBS patients, 91 with 'mild' disease—walking independently but not running, walking 5 m with assistance, or able to stand unaided—were randomized to two plasma exchanges or none. Those receiving therapy began to improve more quickly (4 days versus 8 days), were less likely to deteriorate, and had shorter hospital stays (13 days versus 18 days). While the no-treatment group was slightly worse at 1 year, none of the differences was statistically significant because of the small numbers. Thus, two plasma exchange treatments are recommended in those with 'mild' GBS. The role of IVIG in these 'mild' patients remains unknown, but based on the equivalence in the more severely ill, IVIG treatment seems logical.

The second feature is that Guillain–Barré syndrome is a serious disease with significant mortality and morbidity. For example, in the Plasma Exchange/Sandoglobulin GBS study, mortality averaged 5%. In addition, another 15% of patients were unable to walk independently after 48 weeks.[42] Thus, of 100 patients with severe GBS, approximately 5 will die from the disease and 15 will be unable to walk at 1 year. In addition, quality of life is significantly affected even in those who return to clinical normality.[55] Thus, better treatments are required.

Thirdly, children were excluded from the pivotal treatment studies. While there are anecdotal reports of children improving with IVIG or plasma exchange, it is known that in general children have a more benign course than adults and that their recovery is quicker. Thus, a controlled clinical trial of PE or IVIG in the treatment of children with GBS is needed.

References

1. Landry O. Memoire sur la paralysie du sentiment d'activite musculaire. *Gaz Hopitaux Civils Militaires* 1855; **28**: 269–271.

2. Guillain G, Barré JA, Strohl A. Sur un syndrome de radiculonebrite avec hyperalbuminose du liquide cephalo-rachidien sans reaction cellulaire. Remarques sur les caracteres cliniques et graphiques des reflexes tendineux. *Bull Soc Med Hop Paris* 1916; **40**: 1462.

3. Schonberger LB, Bregman DJ, Sullivan-Bolyai JZ et al. Guillain–Barré syndrome following vaccination in the national influenza immunization program, United States, 1976–1977. *Am J Epidemiol* 1979; **110**: 105–123.

4. Asbury AK, Arnason BG, Karp HR, McFarlin DE. Criteria for diagnosis of Guillain–Barré syndrome. *Ann Neurol* 1978; **3**: 565–566.

5. McLeod JG. Electrophysiological studies in the Guillain–Barré syndrome. *Ann Neurol* 1981; **9** (**suppl**): 20–27.

6. Cornblath DR. Electrophysiology in Guillain–Barré syndrome. *Ann Neurol* 1990; **27** (**suppl**): S17–S20

7. Asbury AK, Arnason BG, Adams RD. The inflammatory lesion in idiopathic polyneuritis. *Medicine* 1969; **48**: 173–215.
8. Haymaker W, Kernohan JW. The Landry–Guillain–Barré syndrome. A clinicopathologic report of fifty fatal cases and a critique of the literature. *Medicine* 1949; **28**: 59–141.
9. Prineas JW. Acute idiopathic polyneuritis. An electron microscope study. *Lab Invest* 1972; **26**: 133–147.
10. Feasby TE, Gilbert JJ, Brown WF et al. An acute axonal form of Guillain–Barré polyneuropathy. *Brain* 1986; **109**: 1115–1126.
11. McKhann GM, Cornblath DR, Ho TW et al. Clinical and electrophysiological aspects of acute paralytic disease of children and young adults in northern China. *Lancet* 1991; **338**: 593–597.
12. McKhann GM, Cornblath DR, Griffin JW et al. Acute motor axonal neuropathy: a frequent cause of acute flaccid paralysis in China. *Ann Neurol* 1993; **33**: 333–342.
13. Ho TW, Mishu B, Li CY et al. Guillain–Barré syndrome in northern China: relationship to *Campylobacter jejuni* infection and anti-glycolipid antibodies. *Brain* 1995; **118**: 597–605.
14. Griffin JW, Li CY, Ho TW et al. Guillain–Barré syndrome in northern China: the spectrum of neuropathologic changes in clinically defined cases. *Brain* 1995; **118**: 577–595.
15. Griffin JW, Li CY, Macko C et al. Early nodal changes in the acute motor axonal neuropathy pattern of the Guillain–Barré syndrome. *J Neurocytol* 1996; **25**: 33–51.
16. Griffin JW, Li CY, Ho TW et al. Pathology of the motor-sensory axonal Guillain–Barré syndrome. *Ann Neurol* 1996; **39**: 17–28.
17. Ho T, Hsieh S, Nachamkin I et al. Motor nerve terminal degeneration provides a potential mechanism for rapid recovery in acute motor axonal neuropathy after Campylobacter infection. *Neurology* 1997; **48**: 717–724.
18. Ho T, Li C, Cornblath D et al. Patterns of recovery in the Guillain–Barré syndromes. *Neurology* 1997; **48**: 695–700.
19. Monos DS, Papaioakim M, Ho TW et al. Differential distribution of HLA alleles in two forms of Guillain–Barré syndrome. *J Infect Dis* 1997; **176 (suppl 2)**: S180–S182.
20. Sheikh KA, Ho TW, Nachamkin I et al. Molecular mimicry in Guillain–Barré syndrome. *Ann NY Acad Sci* 1998; **845**: 307–321.
21. Sheikh KA, Nachamkin I, Ho TW et al. *Campylobacter jejuni* lipopolysaccharides in Guillain–Barré syndrome: molecular mimicry and host susceptibility. *Neurology* 1998; **51**: 371–378.
22. Feasby TE, Hahn AF, Brown WF et al. Severe axonal degeneration in acute Guillain–Barré syndrome: evidence of two different mechanisms? *J Neurol Sci* 1993; **116**: 185–192.
23. Fisher M. An unusual variant of acute idiopathic polyneuritis (syndrome of ophthalmoplegia ataxia and areflexia). *New Engl J Med* 1956; **255**: 57–65.
24. Ropper AH, Wijdicks EFM, Truax BT. *Guillain–Barré Syndrome*. Philadelphia: FA Davis, 1991.
25. Lu JL, Sheikh KA, Wu HS et al. Physiological-pathological correlation in Guillain–Barré syndrome. *Neurology* 1999; **54**: 33–39.
26. Hadden RDM, Cornblath DR, Hughes RAC

et al. Electrophysiological classification of Guillain–Barré syndrome: clinical associations and outcome. *Ann Neurol* 1998; **44**: 780–788.

27. Rees JH, Soudain SE, Gregson NA, Hughes RA. *Campylobacter jejuni* infection and Guillain–Barré syndrome. *New Engl J Med* 1995; **333**: 1374–1379.

28. Meulstee J, van der Meché FGA, Dutch Guillain–Barré Study Group. Electrodiagnostic criteria for polyneuropathy and demyelination: application in 135 patients with Guillain–Barré syndrome. *J Neurol Neurosurg Psych* 1995; **59**: 482–486.

29. Wu H-S, Liu TC, Lu ZL et al. A prospective clinical and electrophysiologic survey of acute flaccid paralysis in Chinese children. *Neurology* 1997; **49**: 1723–1724.

30. Guiloff RJ. Peripheral nerve conduction in Miller Fisher syndrome. *J Neurol Neurosurg Psych* 1977; **40**: 801–807.

31. Alam TA, Chaudhry V, Cornblath DR. Electrophysiological studies in Guillain–Barré syndrome: distinguishing subtypes by published criteria. *Muscle Nerve* 1998; **21**: 1275–1279.

32. Cornblath DR, Mellits ED, Griffin JW et al. Motor conduction studies in the Guillain–Barré syndrome: description and prognostic value. *Ann Neurol* 1988; **23**: 354–359.

33. Meulstee J, van der Meché FGA, Kleyweg RP et al. Prognostic value of electrodiagnosis in the Dutch Guillain–Barré study. *Eur J Neurol* 1995; **2**: 558–565.

34. Ho TW, McKhann GM, Griffin JW. Human autoimmune neuropathies. *Annu Rev Neurosci* 1998; **21**: 187–226.

35. Hartung HP, Pollard JD, Harvey GK, Toyka KV. Immunopathogenesis and treatment of the Guillain–Barré syndrome—Part I. *Muscle Nerve* 1995; **18**: 137–153.

36. Rostami AM. Guillain–Barré syndrome: clinical and immunological aspects. *Springer Seminars in Immunopathology* 1995; **147**: 29–42.

37. Waksman BH, Adams RD. Allergic neuritis: experimental disease in rabbits induced by the injection of peripheral nervous tissue and adjuvants. *J Exp Med* 1955; **102**: 213–235.

38. Waksman BH, Adams RD. A comparative study of experimental allergic neuritis in the rabbit, guinea pig, and mouse. *J Neuropathol Exp Neurol* 1956; **15**: 293–313.

39. Guillain–Barré Study Group. Plasmapheresis and acute Guillain–Barré syndrome. *Neurology* 1985; **35**: 1096–1104.

40. French Cooperative Group on Plasma Exchange in Guillain–Barré Syndrome. Efficacy of plasma exchange in Guillain–Barré syndrome: role of replacement fluids. *Ann Neurol* 1987; **22**: 753–761.

41. Van der Meché FGA, Schmitz PIM, Dutch Guillain–Barré Study Group. A randomized trial comparing intravenous immune globulin and plasma exchange in Guillain–Barré syndrome. *New Engl J Med* 1992; **326**: 1123–1129.

42. Plasma Exchange/Sandoglobulin Guillain–Barré Syndrome Trial Group. Randomised trial of plasma exchange, intravenous immunoglobulin, and combined treatments in Guillain–Barré syndrome. *Lancet* 1997; **349**: 225–230.

43. Hafer-Macko C, Sheikh KA, Li CY et al. Immune attack on the Schwann cell surface in acute inflammatory demyelinating

polyneuropathy. *Ann Neurol* 1996; **39**: 625–635.

44. Hafer-Macko C, Hsieh ST, Li CY et al. Acute motor axonal neuropathy: an antibody-mediated attack on axolemma. *Ann Neurol* 1996; **40**: 635–644.

45. Yuki N. Pathogenesis of axonal Guillain–Barré syndrome: hypothesis. *Muscle Nerve* 1994; **17**: 680–682.

46. Yuki N, Sato S, Tsuji S et al. Frequent presence of anti-GQ1b antibody in Fisher's syndrome. *Neurology* 1993; **43**: 414–417.

47. Willison HJ, Veitch J, Patterson G, Kennedy PGE. Miller Fisher syndrome is associated with serum antibodies to GQ1b ganglioside. *J Neurol Neurosurg Psych* 1993; **56**: 204–206.

48. Chiba A, Kusunoki S, Shimizu T, Kanazawa I. Serum IgG antibody to ganglioside GQ1b is a possible marker of Miller Fisher syndrome. *Ann Neurol* 1992; **31**: 677–679.

49. Carpo M, Pedotti R, Lolli F et al. Clinical correlate and fine specificity of anti-GQ1b antibodies in peripheral neuropathy. *J Neurol Sci* 1998; **155**: 186–191.

50. Chiba A, Kusunoki S, Obata H et al. Serum anti-GQ1b antibody is associated with ophthalmoplegia in Miller Fisher syndrome and Guillain–Barré syndrome: clinical and immunohistochemical studies. *Neurology* 1993; **43**: 1911–1917.

51. Kleyweg RP, van der Meche FG, Meulstee J. Treatment of Guillain–Barré syndrome with high-dose gammaglobulin. *Neurology* 1988; **38**: 1639–1641.

52. Irani DN, Cornblath DR, Chaudhry V et al. Relapse in Guillain–Barré syndrome following treatment with human immune globulin. Neurology 1993; **43**: 872–875.

53. Castro LHM, Ropper AH. Human immune globulin infusion in Guillain–Barré syndrome: worsening during and after treatment. *Neurology* 1993; **43**: 1034–1036.

54. French Cooperative Group on Plasma Exchange in Guillain–Barré Syndrome. Appropriate number of plasma exchanges in Guillain–Barré syndrome. *Ann Neurol* 1997; **41**: 298–306.

55. Bernsen RAJAM, Jacobs HM, de Jager AEJ, van der Meché FGA. Residual health status after Guillain–Barré syndrome. *J Neurol Neurosurg Psych* 1997; **62**: 637–640.

Myasthenia gravis and the Lambert–Eaton myasthenic syndrome

John Newsom-Davis

7

> AChR: acetylcholine receptor; 3,4-DAP: 3,4-diaminopyridine; Ig: immunoglobulin; IVIG: intravenous immunoglobulin; LEMS: Lambert–Eaton myasthenic syndrome; MG: myasthenia gravis; PE: plasma exchange; SCLC: small cell lung cancer; VGCC: voltage-gated calcium channel

Introduction

Ion channels at the neuromuscular junction are the prime targets for autoantibodies in both myasthenia gravis (MG) and the Lambert–Eaton myasthenic syndrome (LEMS). Their vulnerability is likely to arise because of their extracellular domains and the fact that the neuromuscular junction lacks the protection of the blood–nerve barrier. This allows ready access to circulating pathogenic antibodies but, conversely, from the therapeutic standpoint may facilitate the response to agents that reduce or inactivate them.

In MG antibodies reduce the number of postsynaptic muscle acetylcholine receptors (AChRs) either by direct binding, or through an intracellular mechanism ('seronegative MG') as discussed below. The targets in LEMS are presynaptic neuronal voltage-gated calcium channels (VGCCs).

Both of these disorders can occur in paraneoplastic forms. Thymoma is present in 10% of MG patients. Small cell lung cancer associates with LEMS in 60% of patients, and there may also be a weak association with lymphoma.

This chapter reviews the pathophysiology, diagnosis and existing treatments for both of these conditions, with special emphasis on intravenous immunoglobulin therapy.

Myasthenia gravis
Pathophysiology

The fatiguable muscle weakness that characterizes MG is due to the loss of functional AChRs. In the majority (85%) of patients, serum anti-AChR antibodies can be detected, although the titres vary substantially between individuals. Immunoglobulin G (IgG) antibodies to AChRs lead to their loss by varying combinations of complement-mediated lysis, cross-linking of adjacent channels and their consequent down-regulation, and pharmacological block. These antibodies are essentially specific for MG. The antibodies are produced in the thymus gland of patients with early onset (<40 years) MG in which the thymus typically shows follicular hyperplasia, but they are also produced in peripheral blood, bone marrow and lymph nodes. Within individuals the serum antibody titre correlates with disease severity, but this correlation is weak across individuals.

In seronegative MG, there is no doubt that the effector mechanism is also antibody-mediated, as shown by the benefits of plasma exchange, by the passive transfer of the pathophysiological effects of patients' immunoglobulins by injection into mice, and by the observation that 'seronegative' mothers may bear babies with neonatal MG. Research indicates that these patients have serum antibodies to muscle membrane determinants other than the AChR, which lead to AChR inactivation possibly through a second messenger system that induces receptor phosphorylation. These antibodies may in some cases be of IgM class. Phenotypically, the patients do not seem to differ from 'seropositive MG', except that the thymus does not usually show the changes of thymic hyperplasia and, in the author's experience, thymoma is exceptionally rare. About 50% of patients with restricted ocular MG are in the seronegative group.

Diagnosis

The diagnosis is made on clinical grounds, by the detection of serum anti-AChR antibodies or, in seronegative patients, by electromyographic changes (increased decrement and/or jitter) and, where these procedures are not available, by the response to anticholinesterase medication.

Treatment

Most patients improve with anticholinesterase medication, but the benefits diminish progressively as the severity of the underlying disease increases. Overdosage can lead to the downregulation of AChRs and to the risk of cholinergic crisis. Further treatment is indicated in patients who are still significantly weak despite optimal anticholinesterase therapy.

Thymectomy is indicated in those with thymoma (to prevent local spread) and in those who first develop symptoms of MG under the age of 40–45 years. In the latter group, remission can be expected in about 25%, and improvement in a further 50%, developing mainly in the first postoperative year. There is no convincing evidence that myasthenic symptoms improve following thymoma excision.

In those who have failed to respond to thymectomy or for whom it is not indicated, immunosuppressive drug treatment needs to be considered. Corticosteroids have been used for many years, and there is strong clinical evidence for its efficacy in many patients, even though it has not been compared with anticholinesterase therapy alone in a randomized controlled trial. However, adverse effects can be severe, and initiation of treatment can precipitate a severe exacerbation. A recent randomized trial that compared prednisolone alone with prednisolone and azathioprine (2.5 mg/kg body weight) showed that the combination was more effective and better tolerated, allowing prednisolone withdrawal without return of symptoms in about 60% of patients at 3 years.[2]

Plasmapheresis and intravenous immunoglobulin

Plasmapheresis (plasma exchange, PE) was first introduced in the treatment of MG in 1976.[3] Its benefits in the management of myasthenic crisis, and in inducing short-term improvement, have been documented in a number of reports.[4,5] Typically improvement develops 2–3 days after starting the exchange and reaches its maximum about 48 hours after the last exchange of the course. Without coincident immunosuppression, there is a risk of a rebound increase in weakness about 4–5 weeks later. Plasmapheresis is not free of adverse effects. These can include problems with venous access, haemorrhage, postural hypotension and the effects of fluid overload. The procedure is also time-consuming and costly.

Intravenous immunoglobulin (IVIG) was

first reported in the English literature in 1984 in the treatment of MG by Gajdos et al[6] and Arsura et al,[7] but it was some time before it came into more general use. Cosi et al[8] used 0.4 g/kg daily for 5 days to treat 37 patients who had all received additional treatment (immunosuppressive drug treatment and/or thymectomy). The majority of patients improved. Early experience with IVIG was reviewed in 1994 by Edan and Landgraf (who included 10 patients that they themselves had studied).[9] Benefit was documented in 78% of patients overall, but the authors pointed out the need for controlled studies.

The first randomized controlled study was reported by Gajdos et al in 1997.[10] They compared PE (removal of 1.5 × plasma volume) for 3 days with IVIG (0.4 g/kg per day) either for 3 days or 5 days in a group of 87 MG patients. Seventy-two per cent of patients had detectable anti-AChR antibodies and in the remainder the diagnosis was established by standard electromyographic criteria and the response to anticholinesterase medication. About half the patients had undergone previous thymectomy, one third were receiving corticosteroids and about a quarter were receiving azathioprine.

The indication for entry was an exacerbation of myasthenic symptoms. The primary end-point was the change in muscle score from randomization to day 15. The muscle score included measures of limb, trunk and bulbar muscles. There was no significant difference between PE for 3 days and IVIG for 3 days, the two plots being virtually superimposed. Curiously, patients receiving IVIG for 5 days fared rather less well, although their response did not differ significantly from the other two groups. Sixty-six per cent of patients improved in the PE group, 61% in the 3 day IVIG group and 39% in the 5 day IVIG group. The speed of response was greater in the PE group. No information is currently available on the duration of the response, or on the long-term indications for these therapies.

Adverse events

In the study by Gajdos et al, adverse events were more frequent in the PE group (20%), and in two patients they were serious (femoral vein thrombosis and retroperitoneal haematoma).[10] Adverse effects occurred in 2% of the IVIG group. However, cerebral venous thrombosis has been reported following IVIG treatment in MG,[11] and several complications of IVIG treatment have been recognized in other disorders including aseptic meningitis and renal failure.

Mode of action

In seropositive MG, PE appears to act by removal of circulating anti-AChR antibodies, as judged by the decline in titre and associated increase in muscle strength. Seroegative MG also responds to PE, presumably by a similar mechanism.

The mode of action of IVIG is unclear. Liblau et al[12] found that IVIG could in some cases inhibit binding of anti-AChR antibodies in vitro, but whether this is the mechanism in vivo remains to be determined. Findings in the Lambert–Eaton myasthenic syndrome, discussed below, are relevant in this context.

Choice of treatment

Are PE and IVIG of equal effectiveness? The randomized trial described above seems to indicate this, but the rather less good response of the 5 day IVIG group is puzzling (although a chance effect cannot be ruled out). One way of comparing the two treatments is to examine the effects of PE in patients who have failed to respond to IVIG. Stricker et al[13] reported four such patients whose myasthenic crisis (respiratory and bulbar muscle weakness) only improved after PE was introduced. These patients received at least 5 days of each form of treatment. A possible limitation of the Gajdos study[10] is the smaller than usual number of days (3) for which PE was done. However it cannot be confidently concluded, on this evidence, that PE is superior. A late effect of the IVIG treatment, for example, might have been responsible.

In the management of severe myasthenic weakness, the author has a preference for PE (5 day course) because the mode of action is apparent, the response is faster, and perhaps more predictable. Against that view must be set the advantages offered by IVIG with regard to ease of administration, fewer adverse effects (particularly if PE is not in regular use which perhaps makes them more likely), and potential benefits in controlling infection. In those failing to respond to IVIG, PE should be considered.

Lambert–Eaton myasthenic syndrome

Pathophysiology

Lambert–Eaton myasthenic syndrome (LEMS) is characterized by proximal muscle weakness and depressed tendon reflexes which can show prominent post-tetanic potentiation. In addition, there are autonomic changes including dry mouth, constipation and erectile failure in men. About 60% of patients have an associated small cell lung cancer (SCLC). LEMS is a presynaptic disorder in which there is a reduction in the calcium-dependent quantal release of acetylcholine. Typically, a nerve action potential induces the release of 30 or more quanta at each neuromuscular junction in humans, but in LEMS the number may be 10 or fewer.

Passive transfer and other experimental studies have shown that the disorder is caused by antibodies to P/Q type voltage-gated calcium channels (VGCCs).[15] The antibodies lead to VGCC downregulation by cross-linking, thereby reducing calcium influx during nerve-terminal depolarization. They also appear to underlie the autonomic dysfunction.[16] Anti-P/Q type VGCC antibodies can be detected in over 90% of patients by radioimmunoassay using ^{125}I-Conotoxin MVIIC, a specific ligand for these channels.[17] In those with small cell lung cancer, the antibodies appear to be provoked by VGCCs expressed by the tumour. The immune stimulus in noncancer cases is unknown.

Diagnosis

Electromyography shows a greatly reduced amplitude of the compound muscle action potential (measured with surface electrodes) that increases markedly (by 50–1000%) following 10 seconds maximal voluntary contraction, thus differing from MG. However, as in MG, there may be a decrement at slow stimulation rates (3 Hz), and an increase in jitter on single-fibre electromyography. Detection of anti-P/Q type VGCC antibodies is essentially specific for LEMS, and will be positive in over 90% of patients, regardless of whether they have an associated lung cancer.[17] In those in whom a lung cancer is suspected (because of a history of smoking), it should be kept in mind that LEMS may appear up to 5 years before there is radiological evidence of tumour.[14] Regular chest scans will be needed in this group.

Treatment

Both the cancer-associated and noncancer forms of the disorder will be helped by 3,4-diaminopyridine (3,4-DAP), a preparation that blocks voltage-gated potassium channels, thereby prolonging the action potential at the nerve terminal and increasing the number of quanta released.[18] In adults, doses of 20 mg four or five times daily can produce a striking improvement. Excessive dosage can cause epilepsy, and 3,4-DAP is thus contraindicated in patients with a history of epilepsy.

In the SCLC-LEMS group, specific tumour therapy can lead to improvement or remission of the neurological disorder, presumably by reducing antigenic driving of the autoantibody response.[19] There is also evidence that survival may be prolonged in SCLC-LEMS compared with SCLC alone.[20]

In both forms of the disorder, prednisolone may lead to improvement, and in the noncancer group azathioprine or cyclosporin may be indicated in addition.[21]

Plasmapheresis and intravenous immunoglobulin

The response to PE was one of the first features that pointed to an antibody-mediated disease process in LEMS.[22] However, the response is not so dramatic as it often is in MG, and it is slower in developing.

Bird[23] was the first to report clinical and

electrophysiological evidence of improvement following a standard 5 day course of IVIG in a LEMS patient who had no evidence of associated malignancy, but who had the characteristic electromyographic changes. The compound muscle action potential amplitude increased by about 100% following IVIG, and there was a substantial reduction in jitter on single-fibre studies. The patient had previously been successfully treated by PE, but this had had to be abandoned because of problems with venous access. It was concluded that IVIG was as effective as PE in this patient.

Takano et al[24] reported improvement in an SCLC-LEMS patient after IVIG treatment, but ongoing chemotherapy makes it difficult to ascertain the precise role of the IVIG therapy.

Bain et al[25] undertook a randomized, placebo-controlled, double-blind crossover study of IVIG in nine LEMS patients who had no evidence of an underlying cancer. Ongoing treatment with 3,4-DAP, prednisolone and azathioprine continued unchanged. Serial indices of muscle strength (limb strength, vital capacity, drinking time) and the serum titre of anti-P/Q VGCC antibodies were measured at 2-week intervals over an 8-week period following an infusion of 1 g/kg IVIG for 2 consecutive days (total dose 2 g) or of a placebo solution. The wash-out interval was 0–18 weeks. Significant improvements following IVIG infusion were found in each of the three strength measures, values peaking between 2 weeks and 4 weeks. Similarly, there was a decline in the anti-VGCC antibody titre that was most marked between 2 weeks and 4 weeks, and which slowly rose thereafter. In contrast, no consistent change in strength variables nor in the anti-VGCC titre was seen after placebo infusion. The inverse relationship between muscle strength and serum antibody titre suggests that the beneficial effects of treatment, at least in part, result from the lowering of the antibody titre.

Mode of action

The beneficial effect of IVIG treatment in the study by Bain et al[25] does not seem to have been due to a direct antiidiotypic action since the serum anti-VGCC antibody titre was unchanged at 1 week. Moreover, no neutralizing effect of the immunoglobulin could be demonstrated in the binding assay although a late antiidiotypic action cannot be excluded.

Choice of treatment

Although there is circumstantial evidence that PE is effective in LEMS, no randomized trial has been undertaken. IVIG, however, has been clearly shown in a randomized trial to produce short-term improvement that typically lasts 6–8 weeks. It is therefore the treatment of choice in patients with severe weakness, but needs to be coupled with additional long-term treatment. The role of IVIG therapy in the long-term management of LEMS has not been established.

References

1. Newsom-Davis, J. Myasthenia gravis and related syndromes. In: Walton J, Karpati G, Hilton-Jones D, eds. *Disorders of Voluntary Muscle*. Churchill Livingstone: Edinburgh, 1994, 761–780.

2. Palace J, Newsom-Davis J, Lecky B, Myasthenia Gravis Study Group. A randomized double-blind trial of prednisolone alone or with azathioprine in myasthenia gravis. *Neurology* 1998; **50:** 1778–1783.

3. Pinching AJ, Peters DK, Newsom-Davis J. Remission of myasthenia gravis following plasma exchange. *Lancet* 1976; **ii:** 1373–1376.

4. Newsom-Davis J, Vincent A, Wilson S. Long term effects of repeated plasma exchange in myasthenia gravis. *Lancet* 1979; **i:** 464–468.

5. Thornton CA, Griggs RC. Plasma exchange and intravenous immunoglobulin treatment of neuromuscular disease. *Ann Neurol* 1994; **35:** 260–268.

6. Gajdos P, Outin H, Elkharrat D et al. High dose intravenous gammaglobulin for myasthenia gravis. *Lancet* 1984; **i:** 406–407.

7. Arsura EL, Bick A, Brunner NG, Namba T, Grob D. High dose intravenous immunoglobulin in the management of myasthenia gravis. *Arch Intern Med* 1986; **146:** 1365–1368.

8. Cosi V, Lombardi M, Piccolo G, Erbetta A. Treatment of myasthenia gravis with high dose intravenous immunoglobulin. *Acta Neurol Scand* 1991; **84:** 81–84.

9. Edan G, Landgraf F. Experience with intravenous immunoglobulin in myasthenia gravis: a review. *J Neurol Neurosurg Psych* 1994; **57 (suppl):** 55–56.

10. Gajdos P, Chevret S, Clair B et al. Clinical trial of plasma exchange and high dose intravenous immunoglobulin in myasthenia gravis. *Ann Neurol* 1997; **41:** 789–796.

11. Steg RE, Lefkowitz DM. Cerebral infarction following intravenous immunoglobulin therapy for myasthenia gravis. *Neurology* 1994; **44:** 1180–1181.

12. Liblau R, Gajdos P, Bustarret FA et al. Intravenous gammaglobulin in myasthenia gravis: interaction with anti-acetylcholine receptor autoantibodies. *J Clin Immunol* 1991; **11:** 128–131.

13. Stricker RB, Kwiatkowski BJ, Habis JA, Kiprov DD. Myasthenic crisis: response to plasmapheresis following failure of intravenous gammaglobulin. *Arch Neurol* 1993; **50:** 837–840.

14. O'Neill, JH, Murray NM, Newsom-Davis J. The Lambert–Eaton myasthenic syndrome: a review of 50 cases. *Brain* 1988; **111:** 577–596.

15. Lang B, Newsom-Davis J. Immunopathology of the Lambert–Eaton myasthenic syndrome. *Springer Seminars in Immunopathology* 1995; **17:** 3–15.

16. Waterman SA, Lang B, Newsom-Davis J. Effect of Lambert–Eaton myasthenic syndrome antibodies on autonomic neurons in the mouse. *Ann Neurol* 1997; **42:** 147–156.

17. Motomura M, Johnston I, Lang B et al. An improved diagnostic assay for Lambert–Eaton myasthenic syndrome. *J Neurol Neurosurg Psych* 1995; **58:** 85–87.

18. MacEvoy KM, Windebank AJ, Daube JR, Low PA. 3,4-Diaminopyridine in the treatment of Lambert–Eaton myasthenic syndrome. *New Engl J Med* 1989; **321**: 1567–1571.

19. Chalk CH, Murray NMF, Newsom-Davis J et al. Response of the Lambert–Eaton myasthenic syndrome to treatment of associated small-cell lung carcinoma. *Neurology* 1990; **40**: 1552–1556.

20. Maddison P, Newsom-Davis J, Mills KR, Souhami RL. Favourable prognosis in Lambert–Eaton myasthenic syndrome and small-cell lung carcinoma. *Lancet* 1999; **353**: 117–118.

21. Newsom-Davis J, Murray NMF. Plasma exchange and immunosuppressive drug treatment in the Lambert–Eaton myasthenic syndrome. *Neurology* 1984; **34**: 480–485.

22. Lang B, Newsom-Davis J, Wray D et al. Autoimmune aetiology for myasthenic (Eaton–Lambert) syndrome. *Lancet* 1981; **ii**: 224–226.

23. Bird SJ. Clinical and electrophysiologic improvement in Lambert–Eataon syndrome with intravenous immunoglobulin therapy. *Neurology* 1992; **42**: 1422–1423.

24. Takano H, Tanaka M, Koike R et al. Effect of intravenous immunoglobulin in Lambert–Eaton myasthenic syndrome with small cell lung cancer; correlation with the titer of anti-voltage-gated calcium channel antibody. *Muscle Nerve* 1994; **17**: 1073–1075.

25. Bain PG, Motomura M, Newsom-Davis J et al. Effects of intravenous immunoglobulin on muscle weakness and calcium channel autoantibodies in the Lambert–Eaton myasthenic syndrome. *Neurology* 1996; **47**: 678–683.

Relapsing–remitting multiple sclerosis

Franz Fazekas

8

> AIMS: Austrian Immunoglobulin in Multiple Sclerosis [trial]; EDSS: expanded disability status scale; ESS: environmental status scale; IFN: interferon; ISS: incapacity status scale; IVIG: intravenous immunoglobulin; MRI: magnetic resonance imaging; MS: multiple sclerosis

Introduction

Multiple sclerosis (MS) is the most common demyelinating disorder of the central nervous system. Characterized by repeated episodes of neurologic dysfunction or chronically progressing symptoms, it affects primarily young and middle-aged individuals. In central and northern Europe, the northern parts of the USA and Canada prevalence rates range as high as 80–120 patients per 100 000 inhabitants, with women being almost twice as often affected as men. Therefore MS is a major cause of disability of the working population.[1,2] The exact pathophysiologic cascade that leads to the development of MS is not yet fully understood. Certainly, autoimmune mechanisms play a leading role in the attack on brain tissue which is associated with focal inflammation, oedema, demyelination and axonal damage. Tissue destruction is followed by attempts at remyelination and gliosis, leaving areas of focal hardening of the brain which have given the name to this disorder.[3]

For a long time therapeutic interventions in MS were limited to symptomatic treatment of neurologic deficits, and testing of many long-term regimens including life-style modification did not provide convincing evidence for a disease-modifying effect.[4] It was the introduction of beta-interferons that made MS a treatable disorder. Since then, the field has rapidly expanded as a result of various factors, including the improvement in design and performance of clinical trials, studying larger and more homogeneous groups of patients, better and more standardized measurement techniques for clinical and morphologic outcome variables such as the surrogate markers provided by magnetic resonance imaging (MRI); and an improved understanding of the pathophysiology of MS. Despite this progress, overall treatment success of patients with MS is still far from satisfactory. Only about one third of patients with relapsing–remitting MS respond sufficiently to currently approved therapies and there is little or no evidence for a successful therapeutic intervention in patients with secondary or primary progressive MS. This is probably a consequence of some pathophysiologic inhomogeneity of this disorder[5] and of only a limited number of immune mechanisms which can be modified by interferon beta or glatiramer acetate—another promising agent to influence the course of MS.[6] Therefore, we must try hard to extend our therapeutic armamentarium.

Intravenous immunoglobulin (IVIG) is a possible candidate. As reviewed in other chapters of this book, IVIG has proved efficacious in autoimmune-related neurologic disorders primarily affecting the peripheral nervous system. There is experimental evidence for a variety of immunomodulatory effects, many of which could be important for the evolution of MS. Furthermore, IVIG is easily administered, usually well tolerated and has a reasonable safety profile. Exploratory trials have reported beneficial effects of this drug.[7] However, while stimulating, these studies had to remain inconclusive because they were mostly uncontrolled and comprised only a small number of patients, including different types of the disease.

The Austrian Immunoglobulin in MS (AIMS) study was the first double-blind, placebo-controlled trial to document the positive effect of IVIG on the course of MS.[8] These results were supported by two further trials addressing primarily the effect of IVIG on relapses[9] and on monthly MRI.[10] Together these studies provide some rationale to discuss the use of IVIG for treating MS at present and to outline future directions of research.

The AIMS trial

The AIMS study compared a monthly dosage of 0.15–0.2 g/kg body weight of IVIG with physiologic saline over a period of 2 years in 148 MS patients.[8,11] Patients had to have a history of at least two clearly identified and documented relapses during the previous 2 years and a baseline score on Kurtzke's expanded disability status scale (EDSS)[12] of between 1.0 (minor neurological signs without disability) and 6.0 (ambulatory with assistance). Patients were stratified with regard to centre, age, sex and deterioration rate by a centralized, computer-generated randomization schedule. Primary outcome measures were the between-group differences in the absolute change of the EDSS score and in the proportion of patients who improved, remained stable, or worsened in disability, as defined by an increase or a decrease of at least 1.0 grade of the EDSS score by the end of the study. Secondary outcome measures were the number of relapses, the annual relapse rate, the proportion of relapse-free patients, and the time until first relapse during the study period. Sixty-four patients in the IVIG group and 56 in the placebo group completed 2 years of treatment and demographic variables and disease characteristics were well balanced between both treatment groups.

IVIG treatment had a beneficial effect on the course of clinical disability in all analyses. *Table 8.1* compares the change in EDSS score between treatment arms during the study. There was an improvement of one grade or more on the EDSS score in 23 (31%) IVIG-treated patients compared with 10 (14%) placebo-group patients. By contrast, deterioration of disability occurred in 12 (16%) IVIG-treated patients and in 17 (23%) patients of the placebo group ($p = 0.041$). The number of relapses in IVIG-treated patients was about half that in the placebo group (62 versus 116). This resulted in a significantly higher proportion of relapse-free patients receiving IVIG (53% versus 26%; $p = 0.03$). There was an overall 59% reduction of the annual relapse rate in IVIG-treated patients compared to placebo (*Table 8.1*).

Positive treatment effects on disability and the occurrence of relapses were already noted after 6 months of treatment.[11] Moreover, a beneficial effect could also be substantiated by patient self-rating of various items of daily and social living.[13] *Tables 8.2* and *8.3* show the mean changes on items of the incapacity status scale (ISS) and the environmental status scale (ESS) proposed by the International Federation of Multiple Sclerosis Societies.[14] Mean rating scores of 8 of 16 items on the ISS improved in IVIG-treated patients compared with only one area of improvement in the placebo group, and the total mean change of

Table 8.1
Disability and relapses following IVIG treatment in the Austrian Immunoglobulin in Multiple Sclerosis trial.[8]

	IVIG (n = 75)	Placebo (n = 73)	p
Disability			
Baseline EDSS score	3.33 (3.01 to 3.65)	3.97 (2.96 to 3.76)	0.99
Final EDDS score	3.09 (2.72 to 3.46)	3.49 (3.06 to 3.92)	0.008
Change in EDDS score	−0.23 (−0.43 to −0.03)	0.12 (−0.13 to 0.37)	0.008
Annual relapse rate			
Prestudy	1.30 (1.09 to 1.51)	1.41 (1.21 to 1.61)	0.4
Study period	0.52 (0.32 to 0.72)	1.26 (0.75 to 1.77)	0.0037
Year 1	0.49 (0.29 to 0.69)	1.30 (0.79 to 1.81)	0.011
Year 2*	0.42 (0.24 to 0.60)	0.83 (0.59 to 1.07)	0.006

Data are mean (95% CI). EDSS: expanded disability status scale.
*IVIG (n = 65), placebo (n = 63).

all ISS items was significantly better in IVIG than in the placebo group ($p = 0.01$). Better ratings following IVIG treatment were also more frequently noted on the ESS. However, the difference in the total mean change in ESS rating scores between groups did not reach statistical significance.[13] During the study period, the number of patients admitted to hospital (19 IVIG, 28 placebo, $p = 0.06$) and the mean number of days spent in hospital for all patients (3.4 ± 7.6 IVIG, 7.8 ± 14.2 placebo, $p = 0.066$) were lower in IVIG-treated patients, but these differences only approached significance.

IVIG in MS study on relapses

Achiron et al examined the effects of IVIG on relapses in 20 MS patients compared with a similar group of patients receiving physiologic saline.[9] The treatment regimen consisted of a starting dose of 0.4 g/kg body weight per day for 5 consecutive days followed by subsequent IVIG boosters of 0.4 g/kg body weight once daily every 2 months. Secondary outcome measures were exacerbation severity, neurologic disability and a brain MRI score.

IVIG-treated patients experienced a significant drop of the annual exacerbation rate both in the first and second year of the study and these rates were significantly lower

Table 8.2
Treatment effect on incapacity status scale rating.[13] Negative change in score indicates worsening, positive change in score indicates improvement.

	IVIG (64 patients)	Placebo (56 patients)
Climbing stairs	−0.06 ± 0.69	−0.23 ± 0.79
Walking	−0.09 ± 0.50	−0.18 ± 0.83
Transfer to toilet/armchair/bed	−0.14 ± 0.64	−0.16 ± 0.68
Bowel function	0.06 ± 0.83	0.04 ± 0.60
Bladder function	0.17 ± 1.25	−0.14 ± 0.64
Bathing	−0.08 ± 0.63	−0.07 ± 0.71
Dressing	−0.02 ± 0.52	−0.16 ± 0.63
Personal hygiene	−0.03 ± 0.31	−0.14 ± 0.75
Eating	−0.05 ± 0.33	−0.07 ± 0.66
Vision	0.11 ± 0.51	0.04 ± 0.60
Speaking, hearing	0.31 ± 0.31	−0.04 ± 0.47
Need for general medical assistance	0.06 ± 0.61	−0.07 ± 0.63
Mood	0.23 ± 0.85	−0.13 ± 0.67
Intellectual performance	0.05 ± 0.60	−0.16 ± 0.73
Fatigue ability	0.09 ± 0.73	−0.21 ± 0.85
Sexuality	−0.29 ± 1.18	−0.32 ± 1.59

Table 8.3
Treatment effect on environmental status scale rating.[13] Negative change in score indicates worsening, positive change in score indicates improvement.

	IVIG (64 patients)	Placebo (56 patients)
Performance at work	−0.50 ± 1.46	−0.52 ± 1.49
Financial/economic situation	0.13 ± 0.58	−0.02 ± 0.62
Housing	0.11 ± 0.74	−0.16 ± 1.01
Need for assistance in daily living	−0.08 ± 0.84	−0.21 ± 0.78
Mobility/transportation	−0.05 ± 0.74	−0.13 ± 0.81
Need for social services	0.16 ± 0.72	−0.13 ± 0.38
Participation in social activities	0.08 ± 0.90	−0.16 ± 0.99

Table 8.4
Effect of IVIG treatment on relapses as observed by Achiron et al.[9]

Annual relapse rate	IVIG (n = 20)	Placebo (n = 20)	p
Prestudy	1.85 ± 0.26	1.55 ± 0.17	0.34
Study period	0.59	1.61	0.0006
Year 1	0.75 ± 0.16*	1.8 ± 0.2	0.0002
Year 2	0.42 ± 0.14*	1.42 ± 0.23	0.0009

*$p < 0.05$ compared with baseline.

than those of placebo-treated patients (*Table 8.4*). The number of exacerbation-free patients was also significantly higher following medication with IVIG during both years (6 versus 0, $p = 0.001$) and Kaplan–Meier analysis of the probability of remaining exacerbation-free during the 2-year study period was significantly in favour of IVIG. There was a trend towards reduced neurologic disability in the IVIG group compared with a minor increase of the EDSS score in placebo-treated patients. Improvement by at least one point on the EDSS score was noted in 24% of patients following IVIG treatment compared with 11% in the placebo group, whereas 14% of patients deteriorated on IVIG compared with 17% on placebo ($p = 0.03$). The mean MRI scores generated from the number and diameter of demyelinating plaques were not significantly different between the two treatment arms at the end of the second year, but data for only 30 individuals were available for this type of analysis.[9,15]

IVIG and monthly MRI

A crossover study of 26 patients with relapsing–remitting or secondary progressive MS with relapses examined the effect of IVIG on disease activity using frequent gadolinium-enhanced MRI.[10] IVIG treatment consisted of the administration of 2 g/kg body weight over 2 consecutive days at monthly intervals. In a randomized fashion, one group of patients was first treated with IVIG for 6 months and after a 3-month wash-out period was switched over to another 6 months of placebo treatment. The other group of patients was treated in reverse order.

IVIG significantly reduced the mean number of new and of all gadolinium-enhanced lesions by approximately 60%

Table 8.5
Monthly number of gadolinium-enhancing lesions following high-dose IVIG: Intention-to-treat analysis (n=21).[10]

	Baseline*	IVIG	Placebo	p
All lesions	3.6 ± 7.7	1.3 ± 2.3	2.9 ± 5.4	0.003
New lesions	3.6 ± 7.7	1.1 ± 2.0	2.2 ± 4.2	0.002

*Average of the two baseline scans.

compared with placebo (*Table 8.5*). Disease activity on MRI decreased after 1 month of treatment with IVIG and then remained stable, whereas no significant changes in activity were observed during treatment with placebo. Of the 18 patients who completed the entire crossover study, 37% had one or more active scans on 6-monthly serial MRI during IVIG treatment compared with 68% when receiving placebo ($p < 0.01$). Four of these patients had no gadolinium-enhanced lesions during the whole IVIG treatment period but none was free of new gadolinium-enhanced lesions while on placebo. No significant between-group differences were found in regard to the total T_2 lesion load. A significantly greater number of patients were relapse-free when receiving IVIG than when on placebo medication (15 versus 7, $p = 0.02$). In IVIG treatment periods, the number of relapses was 42% lower when considering those 21 patients who had completed at least 1 month of follow-up and two MRIs in the second treatment period. Also, a greater number of patients improved on IVIG than on placebo. No significant differences were found with regard to changes in the EDSS score between the two treatment periods.

A more detailed comparison of these three trials concerning patient characteristics and the impact of IVIG on disability and relapses has been provided by Fazekas et al.[16] All the studies focused on patients with relapsing–remitting MS. While quite similar populations appear to have been studied in the AIMS trial and by Achiron et al, more aggressive and advanced types of the disease appear to have been included in the trial of Sørensen et al. In this context, it is important to note also that the dosage of IVIG was similar in the first two trials while it was 10 times higher in the frequent MRI study. Throughout these trials, there is a consistent effect concerning the reduction of relapses and a more favourable course of disability following IVIG treatment. This clinical evidence for a reduction of disease activity is confirmed by the drop in new and contrast-enhancing lesions on monthly MRI. Furthermore, patient self-reporting of activities of daily and social living in the AIMS trial attests to the positive effect of IVIG on various aspects of life that are important for a patient's wellbeing.

Side-effects were rarely observed in both the AIMS trial and the study by Achiron et al. These effects consisted of a transient rash, fatigue, headaches and low-grade fever which spontaneously resolved within a few hours. An unexpectedly high number of acute and chronic adverse events in more than 60% of patients were seen in the frequent MRI study by Sørensen et al. Acute adverse events consisted of headaches, nausea and urticarial rashes. Symptoms were usually mild and could be diminished either by reducing the infusion rate or by administering an antihistaminic drug before the infusion. The most common major chronic side-effect was severe eczema, observed in 11 of 23 patients during treatment with IVIG. In all patients, the eczema eventually resolved after discontinuation of IVIG therapy but in some patients it persisted for several weeks after the last infusion. Differences in the concentration of cytokines between commercially available preparations of IVIG could be one explanation for this unusual adverse effect profile because this problem has not been noted as frequently in other instances of high-dose treatment.[17] In addition, one patient developed hepatitis C and one experienced deep venous thrombosis, which led to death from a pulmonary embolism.

Current implications for the use of IVIG

At present, the AIMS trial appears to provide the most reasonable guidance in regard to which MS patient and what dosage might be considered suitable for treatment with IVIG. So far the AIMS study has been the largest well-controlled clinical trial to investigate the efficacy of IVIG. It showed significant benefit of monthly IVIG therapy in a dosage of 0.15–0.2 g/kg body weight both in regard to the course of disability and the frequency of relapses. This regimen was associated with a low number of side-effects, and its costs are similar or even lower than that of other immunomodulatory drugs that are currently approved for MS. However, there are caveats to consider.

The number of patients successfully treated in the AIMS trial is small in comparison with the large patient experience concerning efficacy of interferon beta. Also, the clinical results of the AIMS study cannot be supported by simultaneously obtained morphologic MRI data. In this context it

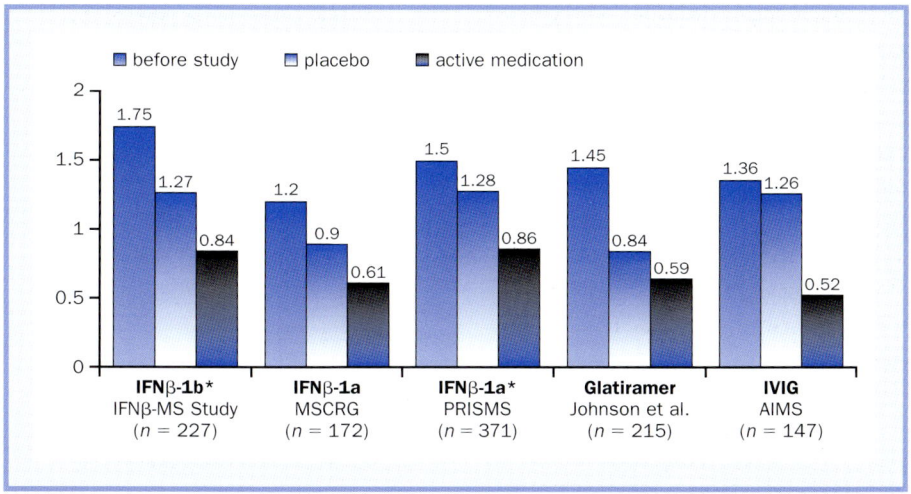

Figure 8.1
Annual relapse rates in trials of different immunomodulatory drugs (adapted from Fazekas et al).[19]
*High-dose treatment groups.

should be mentioned that MRI evidence for a suppression of disease activity has now also been generated for glatiramer acetate.[18] Furthermore, the exact mechanisms by which IVIG—especially in relatively low amounts—can ameliorate the course of MS have not yet been elucidated. Does this leave any indications for the use of IVIG?

There are various reasons to respond positively to this question. The magnitude of treatment effects of IVIG compares favourably with that of other immunomodulatory drugs such as interferon beta and glatiramer acetate (*Fig. 8.1*). The frequency and route of administration of interferon beta and glatiramer acetate, local reactions at the injection site, or continuing other side-effects such as flu-like symptoms, may not be tolerable for some individuals. A significant number of patients fail to respond or stop responding to either interferon beta or glatiramer acetate. Furthermore, there may be conditions under which these drugs should not be given, such as impending pregnancy or breast-feeding. In all these instances, IVIG treatment appears to have potential as a reasonable alternative. Certainly, IVIG should not yet be recommended for other settings.

There is at least anecdotal evidence for the lack of efficacy in more advanced or rapidly progressive MS.[20] Whether effectiveness could then be improved by a higher dosage of IVIG awaits clarification.

References

1. Thompson A, Polman C, Hohlfeld R. *Multiple Sclerosis: Clinical Challenges and Controversies.* London: Martin Dunitz, 1998.

2. Hartung H, Fazekas F, Hohlfeld R. Multiple Sklerose. In: Hopf H, Deuschl G, Diener H et al, eds. *Neurologie in Praxis und Klinik,* 3rd edition. Stuttgart: Thieme, 1999, 909–942.

3. Allen I. Pathology of multiple sclerosis. In: Metthews W, ed. *McAlpine's Multiple Sclerosis,* 2nd edition. Edinburgh: Churchill Livingstone, 1991, 341–378.

4. Thompson A. Multiple sclerosis: symptomatic treatment. *J Neurol* 1996; **243**: 559–565.

5. Lassmann H. Neuropathology in multiple sclerosis: new concepts. *Mult Scler* 1998; **4**: 93–98.

6. Rudick R, Goodkin D. *Multiple Sclerosis Therapeutics.* London: Martin Dunitz, 1999.

7. Sørensen P. Treatment of multiple sclerosis with IVIG: potential effects and methodology of clinical trials. *J Neurol Neurosurg Psych* 1994; **57 (suppl)**: 62–64.

8. Fazekas F, Deisenhammer F, Strasser-Fuchs S et al. Randomised placebo-controlled trial of monthly intravenous immunoglobulin therapy in relapsing–remitting multiple sclerosis. *Lancet* 1997; **349**: 589–593.

9. Achiron A, Gabbay U, Gilad R et al. Intravenous immunoglobulin treatment in multiple sclerosis: effect on relapses. *Neurology* 1998; **50**: 398–402.

10. Sørensen P, Wanscher B, Jensen C et al. Intravenous immunoglobulin G reduces MRI activity in relapsing multiple sclerosis. *Neurology* 1998; **50**: 1273–1281.

11. Fazekas F, Deisenhammer F, Strasser-Fuchs S et al. Treatment effects of monthly intravenous immunoglobulin on patients with relapsing–remitting multiple sclerosis: further analysis of the Austrian Immunoglobulin in MS Study. *Mult Scler* 1997; **3**: 137–141.

12. Kurtzke J. Rating neurologic impairment in multiple sclerosis: an expanded disability status scale (EDSS). *Neurology* 1983; **33**: 1444–1452.

13. Strasser-Fuchs S, Fazekas F, Deisenhammer F et al. The Austrian Immunoglobulin in MS (AIMS) study: final analysis. *Mult Scler* 2000 (in press).

14. International Federation of Multiple Sclerosis Societies. Symposium on a minimal record of disability for multiple sclerosis. Vancouver, Canada, 11–12 September 1983. *Acta Neurol Scand* 1984; **101 (suppl)**: 1–217.

15. Achiron A, Barak Y, Sarova-Pinhas I. Use of intravenous immunoglobulin in multiple sclerosis. *BioDrugs* 1998; **9**: 465–475.

16. Fazekas F, Strasser-Fuchs S, Sørensen P. Intravenous immunoglobulin trials in multiple sclerosis. *Int MS J* 1999; **6**: 14–21.

17. Stangel M, Hartung H, Marx P, Gold R. Side effects of high-dose intravenous immunoglobulins. *Clin Neuropharmacol* 1997; **20**: 385–393.

18. Comi G, Filippi M, for the Copaxone MRI Study Group. The effect of glatiramer acetate (Copaxone) on MRI-detected disease activity in patients with relapsing–remitting multiple sclerosis: a multi-centre, randomised, double-blind, placebo-controlled study extended by open-label treatment [abstract]. *Mult Scler* 1999; **5 (suppl 1)**: S20.

19. Fazekas F, Strasser-Fuchs S, Gold R, Hartung H. Intravenous immunoglobulin. In: Rudick R, Goodkin D, eds. *Multiple Sclerosis Therapeutics*. London: Martin Dunitz, 1999, 309–322.

20. Francis GS, Freedman MS, Antel JP. Failure of intravenous immunoglobulin to arrest progression of multiple sclerosis: a clinical and MRI based study. *Mult Scler* 1997; **3**: 370–376.

Neuro-Behçet syndrome

Aksel Siva and Ayşe Altıntaş

BD: Behçet's disease; CNS: central nervous system; CSF: cerebrospinal fluid; CT: computerized tomography; EDSS: expanded disability status scale; EMG: electromyography; IFN: interferon; IL: interleukin; IVIG: intravenous immunoglobulin: MRI: magnetic resonance imaging; NBS: neuro-Behçet syndrome; pNBS: parenchymal NBS; TNF: tumour necrosis factor; VST: venous sinus thrombosis

Behçet's disease

Behçet's disease (BD) is a multisystem vascular-inflammatory disease of unknown origin. The classical triad of oral and genital ulcerations with uveitis was originally described by the Turkish dermatologist Hulusi Behçet in 1937.[1] Other systems reported to be involved through the course of the disease are the cardiovascular, pulmonary, gastrointestinal and central nervous systems.[2-4] Currently the most widely used diagnostic criteria are those of the International Study Group's classification, according to which definitive diagnosis requires recurrent oral ulcerations plus two of the following: recurrent genital ulcerations, skin lesions, eye lesions and a positive pathergy test.[5,6]

Despite BD being originally described as a dermatological disease, the major causes of morbidity and mortality result from ocular, major vascular or neurological involvement.[7–9] Arterial and venous large vessel complications (such as pulmonary artery aneurysms, superior or inferior vena cava syndromes) are seen in 25–30% of cases, while a possibly higher proportion may have small vessel involvement including postcapillary venules.[3,10–13] Venous vascular involvement is more common than arterial lesions in Turkish patients.[13]

The epidemiology of the disease shows a geographic variation: BD is seen more commonly along the Silk Route, which extends from the Mediterranean region to Japan.[14] This is coupled by a similar variation in HLA-B51, which is strongly associated with the disease in the high-prevalence areas.[15–18] Despite broadened clinical understanding of this disease, the aetiologic factors remain obscure and speculative; viral agents, immunological factors, genetic causes, bacterial factors and fibrinolytic defects have all been implicated.[19–22] The vessel wall and perivascular mononuclear cell infiltration consistent with vasculitis involving both arterial and venous systems has been shown in histopathologic studies.[3,20,23] It is postulated that a genetic susceptibility, together with a possible trigger by an extrinsic factor such as an infectious agent, is responsible for the observed vasculitis.

Three major pathophysiologic changes have been reported in BD: excessive function of neutrophils, endothelial injury with vasculitis, and autoimmune responses. Histopathologic and immunohistochemical studies of the biopsy lesions obtained from patients with BD reveal typical features of 'vasculitis' with perivascular infiltrations of T lymphocytes, B lymphocytes and neutrophils.[20,22,24] These cells secrete proinflammatory cytokines such as TNFα, IL-1, IFNγ and IL-6, cytokines that may cause vascular endothelial injury and dysfunction.[24–27] The uniformity of such a relationship, however, needs to be confirmed as it has not been studied yet in different clinical forms of BD.

Leucocytosis with neutrophilia and aseptic neutrophilic infiltration into the lesions are characteristic of the active phase of BD. Patients' neutrophils express an enhanced superoxide synthesis[28] and increased level of adhesion molecules, presumably mediating elevated effector functions and facilitating interaction with endothelial cells.[24] The effect of colchicine treatment on neutrophils was related to the therapeutic improvement of symptoms and supports the importance of neutrophils.[29] A significant correlation between the neutrophil hyperfunction and the possession of HLA-B51 phenotype was reported and it was suggested that HLA-51 molecule itself may be responsible, at least in part, for neutrophil hyperfunction in BD.[30] However, we still do not know whether the HLA-B51 or a gene in linkage disequilibrium with HLA-B51 is the predisposing locus for BD. Furthermore in recent years, the possible role of HLA-C locus and MICA gene to induce susceptibility to BD was reported.[18]

Both phenotypical and functional abnormalities of $\gamma\delta$ T cells were detected in BD.[24] These T cells exhibited the characteristic features of memory T cells and expressed a unique CD45RA isoform, 205 kd (memory cell) but not 220 kd (naïve cell), whereas those from normal donors dominantly expressed CD45RO. CD45RA+ $\gamma\delta$ T cells produce much more TNFα and β than do CD45RO+ $\gamma\delta$ T cells from normal individuals. They have similarities with natural killer cells such as producing perforin granules. An accumulation of $\gamma\delta$ T cells has been reported in the peripheral blood of BD patients. This accumulation also can be shown in the cerebrospinal fluid from BD patients with neurologic involvement.[24] These findings suggest that T cells may also play a considerable part in the vascular endothelial injury seen in BD.

Vascular injuries with thrombotic tendency are another characteristic feature of BD.[20,22] The damaged or activated endothelial cells are another stimulator to neutrophils. Abnormalities described as associated with the vascular lesions are the presence of antiendothelial cell antibodies, higher von Willebrand factor antigen levels[22,31–33] and the presence of circulating immune complexes.[34] In addition, circulating proinflammatory cytokines are involved in activating both neutrophils and endothelial cells. Activated endothelial cells secrete adhesion molecules and this facilitates interaction between endothelial cells and neutrophils. These factors form a vicious circle to promote the disease.[24]

Neuro-Behçet syndrome

Neurological involvement in BD, which is not included in the current International Study Group's classification, was first reported in 1941 by Knapp[35] and the term 'neuro-Behçet syndrome' was introduced by Cawara and D'Ermo in 1954.[36] Although the reported range of BD patients developing neurological involvement is 2.2–49%,[9,37,38] this rate does not exceed 10% in large series and was found to be 4.8% in a nonselective series at the Behçet's Disease Research Center of Cerrahpaşa School of Medicine (author's unpublished data).

Neurological complications occur more commonly in men. In 164 well-documented cases (inclusion criteria shown in *Table 9.1*), the male to female ratio was 3.8 : 1, whereas the male to female ratio in the total BD

Table 9.1
Diagnostic criteria for neuro-Behçet syndrome.

A. Fulfilling the international diagnostic criteria for Behçet's disease[5,6]
B. Onset of neurological symptoms otherwise not explained by any other known systemic or neurological disease or treatment
C. Presence of at least one of the following:
  1. Objective abnormalities on neurological examination
  2. Abnormal neuroimaging findings suggestive of NBS
  3. Abnormal cerebrospinal fluid findings suggestive of NBS
  4. Abnormal neurophysiological studies consistent with the current neurological symptoms (EMG; evoked potentials)

population recorded in the research centre was 1.8 : 1. This clearly shows a male predisposition for the evolution of neurological complications in BD, a tendency also observed by other investigators.[9] Such a prominent male dominance has also been observed for other vascular complications of BD. The mean ages at onset of BD and neuro-Behçet syndrome (NBS) were 26.7 ± 8.0 years and 32.0 ± 8.7 years respectively in this series, consistent with other large series.[9,39]

Patients with BD may present with different neurological problems, some directly and some indirectly related to the disease (*Table 9.2*). The most common neurological symptom in the author's practice is headache. A relatively large number of patients referred because of headache have either tension type, migraine or migraine-like headaches. However, some report a severe headache of recent onset not consistent with a primary headache. Whether or not they have any neurological signs, these patients need to be examined carefully as such a symptom may indicate the onset of NBS, in the form of either venous sinus thrombosis or parenchymal central nervous system involvement, the two major neurological complications of BD. Headache is also reported by some patients during acute ocular inflammation.

Besides isolated headache, NBS may present with focal or multifocal central nervous system (CNS) dysfunction with or without headache. The most common symptoms detected at onset in the author's series were headache (61.6%), weakness of upper motor neuron type (53.7%), brainstem and cerebellar symptoms (49%), cognitive and

Table 9.2
The neurological spectrum of Behçet's disease.

> Headache
> Venous sinus thrombosis (extraaxial NBS)
> Central nervous system involvement (intraaxial NBS/parenchymal NBS)
> (Neuro-) Psycho-Behçet syndrome
> Peripheral nervous system involvement
> Complications of BD treatments
> Secondary or coincidental neurological involvement

behavioural changes (16%). As patients with NBS are young and present not infrequently with an acute or subacute brainstem syndrome or hemiparesis, this possibility is often included in the differential diagnosis of multiple sclerosis and stroke of young onset, especially in the absence of the known systemic symptoms and signs. However, in most cases with BD who present with neurological manifestations a careful history will reveal either the presence or a past history of recurrent oral ulcerations with or without other systemic findings of the disease.

Clinical and imaging data suggest that NBS can present with a variety of neurological symptoms which may be classified into two forms, one attributable to small venous disease with focal or multifocal CNS involvement, seen in the majority of patients—parenchymal neuro-Behçet syndrome (pNBS), intraaxial NBS—and the other form due to dural venous sinus thrombosis with limited symptoms and a better prognosis. These two types of involvement have been reported to occur in the same individual in only a very few cases,[39,40] and none has been observed in the author's series. Patients with dural venous sinus thrombosis (VST)—extraaxial NBS—generally have an uncomplicated outcome. It is likely that these two forms have a different pathogenesis, and it is the former group with small vessel inflammation who should be considered for aggressive treatment as a substantial proportion of these patients will have a relapsing–remitting course, with some developing a secondary progressive course later. A few from this group will have progressive CNS dysfunction from the onset.

Rare presentations that were reported include isolated optic neuritis, psychiatric manifestations (neuro-psycho-Behçet syndrome), intracerebral haemorrhage due to ruptured aneurysms, extrapyramidal syndromes and peripheral neuropathy.[41–51]

In the author's series the rate of pNBS was found to be 75.6% and that of VST 12.2% with the remaining subjects having other or indefinite diagnoses. These rates are consistent with other large series.[9]

Imaging studies in parenchymal neuro-Behçet syndrome have shown that brain magnetic resonance imaging (MRI) is both specific and more sensitive than computerized tomography (CT) in demonstration of reversible inflammatory parenchymal lesions. Lesions are generally located within the brainstem, occasionally with extension to the diencephalon, or within the periventricular and subcortical white matters.[52-56] With the exception of the isolated periventricular and subcortical white matter lesions which were rarely seen in our series, the images seen in these patients do not cause any confusion with multiple sclerosis. The imaging findings of pNBS also do not correspond to thrombotic or embolic stroke.

The parenchymal distribution of lesions in pNBS supports the hypothesis of a small vessel vasculitis, mainly of venular involvement, and the known anatomical arrangement of central nervous system intraaxial veins may explain the predominant involvement of the brainstem structures observed radiologically in pNBS.[56] The histopathologic changes reported in parenchymal CNS involvement of the disease cover a wide spectrum that include vasculitis, a low-grade inflammation, demyelination and degenerative changes.[57-59] However, a clear-cut vasculitis is not observed in all cases and there are contradicting reports on the pathology observed in this region.[60,61]

Cerebrospinal fluid studies may show inflammatory changes in most cases with pNBS if performed during the acute stage. A pleocytosis consistent with a dominance of neutrophils over lymphocytes was reported but this was not a uniform finding as a lymphocytic pleocytosis was also observed in some cases.[9,62] A mild to moderate increase of protein was also detected.[62] In a follow-up study the presence of pleocytosis with elevated protein levels at the initial evaluation was found to be associated with a progressive course and worse prognosis.[63] Changes seen in patients with VST remain limited to increased pressure with normal cell count and biochemistry.

Neurological involvement in BD is a remarkable cause of morbidity and approximately half of the patients are moderate to severely disabled after 10 years. Disability was rated in the author's series using a modified form of the expanded disability status scale (EDSS), which is an ordinal scale originally devised for multiple sclerosis-associated disability.[64] It was found that 45.1% of patients (all with CNS–parenchymal involvement) had a disability level on the EDSS of 6 or more (requiring assistance for ambulation) 10 years after the onset of neurological symptoms and signs. Onset with cerebellar symptoms and a progressive course were unfavourable factors, while onset with headache and a diagnosis of VST was favourable (author's unpublished data).

Treatment of NBS

Treatment of acute episodes

Most physicians treat acute CNS involvement with glucocorticoids in BD, but the effects are short-lived and these drugs do not prevent further attacks or progression.[65,66] Attacks of CNS involvement were treated either with oral prednisone (1 mg/kg for 2 weeks) or with high-dose intravenous methylprednisolone (1 g per day for 5–7 days), both followed with oral tapering over 2–3 months. There was no difference between the two regimens but the impression was received that stopping glucocorticoids early was associated with exacerbations in some cases. Spontaneous remission was also observed in two cases in whom glucocorticoids could not be used for various reasons.

Long-term treatment

Although colchicine, some immunosuppressive agents, interferon alpha pentoxyfylline and more recently thalidomide have been shown to be effective in treating some of the systemic manifestations of BD,[22,66,67] no known treatment has been shown to be effective in pNBS in well-conducted placebo-controlled studies.

Chlorambucil was reported to have some efficacy in meningoencephalitis of Behçet's disease,[68] but the number of cases were few and it was a retrospective study. The author's experience with this agent in pNBS although limited was not rewarding and its serious side-effects exclude its use. Treatment with other immunosuppressive drugs such as azathioprine, cyclosporin and cyclophosphamide —either alone or in combination (such as azathioprine with cyclosporin)—for other systemic manifestations of BD, has not been observed to prevent the development of pNBS or its exacerbations or stop its progression.

IVIG treatment

The use of intravenous immunoglobulin (IVIG) in parenchymal NBS was considered because of its various immunologic effects and reports of its efficacy in the treatment of some vasculitic syndromes.[69–73] In theory, IVIG would be expected to have a possible regulatory effect in the reported immunologic abnormalities of BD and pNBS described above, some of these being early effects on the neutralization of circulating autoantibodies, inhibition of complement-mediated damage, changes in solubility and clearance of immune complexes and modulation of production of proinflammatory cytokines such as IL-1, IL-2, IL-6, IFNγ and TNFα.[69]

Only a few cases, however, were treated. One case with progressive CNS involvement showed no improvement. Another patient, a 35-year-old man with a relatively rapid progressive course and severe tetraparesis, deteriorated further within a week after the termination of the IVIG and died after a few weeks. It is not clear if the death of the patient was due to the natural course of the disease or somehow related to the treatment applied. One patient received IVIG treatment in another hospital during a CNS exacerbation without any significant response. Another severe progressive case who did not respond to IVIG was treated at the Istanbul University Medical School (P Serdaroğlu, G Akman-Demir, personal communication). Another two cases of BD showed some improvement after IVIG treatment in Ankara at the Hacettepe Medical School (E Tan, personal communication). One of them was a 38-year-old man who had an attack of hemiparesis, and the other was a 43-year-old woman with a demyelinating polyneuropathy. However, as CNS attacks may show some improvement even without treatment and as clinical polyneuropathy is extremely rare in BD, it is difficult to interpret these results.

In summary, this limited experience does not warrant the use of IVIG in neuro-Behçet syndrome, with the possible exception of patients with Behçet disease who have only well-documented peripheral nerve involvement, unresponsive to other treatments.

References

1. Behçet H. Uber residivierende, aphtöse, durch ein virus verursachte Geschwüre am Mund, am Auge und an den Genitalien. *Derm Wochenschr* 1937; **105**: 1152–1157.

2. Lakhanpal S, Tanı K, Lie JT et al. Pathological features of Behçet's syndrome: a review of Japanese autopsy registry data. *Hum Pathol* 1985; **16**: 790–795.

3. O'Duffy JD. Vasculitis in Behçet's disease. *Rheum Dis Clin North Am* 1990; **16**: 423–431.

4. Yazıcı H, Yurdakul S, Hamuryudan V. Behçet's syndrome. In: Klippel J, Dieppe P, eds. *Rheumatology*. London: Gower Medical, 1997, 7.26.1–6.

5. International Study Group for Behçet's disease. Criteria for diagnosis of Behçet's disease. *Lancet* 1990; **335**: 1078–1080.

6. International Study Group for Behçet's disease. Evaluation of diagnostic (classification) criteria in Behçet's disease—towards internationally agreed criteria. *Br J Rheumatol* 1992; **31**: 299–308.

7. Ben Ezra D, Cohen E. Treatment and visual prognosis in Behçet's disease. *Br J Ophthalmol* 1986; **70**: 589–592.

8. Hamuryudan V, Yurdakul S, Moral F et al. Pulmonary arterial aneurysms in Behçet's syndrome: a report of 24 cases. *Br J Rheumatol* 1994; **33**: 48–51.

9. Serdaroğlu P. Behçet's disease and the nervous system. *J Neurol* 1998; **245**(4): 197–205.

10. James DG, Thompson A. Recognition of the diverse cardiovascular manifestations in Behçet's disease. *Am Heart J* 1982; **103**: 457–458.

11. Clausen J, Bierring F. Involvement of postcapillary venules in Behçet's disease. *Acta Dermatovener* (Stockholm) 1983; **63**: 191–197.

12. Park JH, Han MC, Bettmann MA. Arterial manifestations of Behçet's disease. *AJR* 1984; **143**: 821–825.

13. Koç Y, Güllü I, Akpek G et al. Vascular involvement in Behçet's disease. *J Rheumatol* 1992; **19**: 402–410.

14. Ohno S. Behçet's disease in the world. In: Lehner T, Barnes CG, eds. *Recent Advances in Behçet's Disease*. London: RSM, 1986, 181–186.

15. Yazıcı H, Akhan G, Yalçın B, Müftüoğlu A. The high prevalence of HLA-B5 in Behçet's disease. *Clin Exp Immunol* 1977; **30**: 259–261.

16. Yurdakul S, Günaydın I, Tüzün H et al. The prevalence of Behçet's syndrome in a rural area in Northern Turkey. *J Rheumatol* 1988; **15**: 820–822.

17. Ohno S, Ohguchi M, Hirose S et al. Close association of HLA-BW51 with Behçet's disease. *Arch Ophthalmol* 1982; **100**: 1455–1458.

18. Mizuki N, Inoko H, Ohno S. Molecular genetics (HLA) of Behçet's disease. *Yonsei Med J* 1997; **38(6)**: 333–349.

19. Gamble CN, Wiesner KB, Shapiro RF, Boyer WJ. The immune complex pathogenesis of glomerulonephritis and pulmonary vasculitis in Behçet's disease. *Am J Med* 1979; **66**: 1031–1039.

20. Kansu E. Endothelial cell dysfunction in Behçet's disease. In: Ansell BM, Bacon PA, Lie JT, Yazıcı H, eds. *Vasculitides*. London: Chapman & Hall, 1996, 207–221.

21. Yazıcı H. The place of Behçet's syndrome among the autoimmune diseases. *Int Rev Immunol* 1997; **14**: 1–10.

22. Yazıcı H, Yurdakul V, Hamuryudan V. Behçet's syndrome. *Curr Opin Rheumatol* 1999; **11**: 53–57.

23. Lakhanpal S, O'Duffy JD, Lie JT. Pathology. In: Plotkin GR, Calabro JJ, O'Duffy JD, eds. *Behçet Syndrome. A Contemporary Synopsis*. New York: Future Publishing, 1988, 101–142.

24. Sakane T, Suzuki N, Nagafuchi H. Etiopathology of Behçet's disease: immunological aspects. *Yonsei Med J* 1997; **38(6)**: 350–358.

25. Sakane T, Suzuki N, Takeno M. Innate and acquired immunity in Behçet's disease. *Eighth International Congress on Behçet's Disease*, Reggio Emilia, Oct 1998, abstract, 56.

26. Yamakawa Y, Sugita Y, Nagatani T et al. IL-6 in patients with Behçet's disease. *J Derm Sci* 1996; **11(3)**: 189–195.

28. Mege JL, Dilşen N, Sanguedolce V et al. Overproduction of monocyte derived TNF-α, IL-6, IL-8 and increased neutrophil superoxide generation in Behçet's disease. A comparative study with FMF and healthy subjects. *J Rheumatol Can* 1993; **20(9)**: 1544–1549.

29. Yasui K, Ohta K, Kabayashi M et al. Successful treatment of Behçet's disease with pentoxifylline. *Ann Intern Med* 1996; **124**: 891–893.

30. Takeno M, Kariyone A, Yamashita N et al. Excessive function of peripheral blood neutrophils from patients with Behçet's

31. Direskeneli H, Keser G, D'Cruz D et al. Anti-endothelial cell antibodies, endothelial proliferation and von Willebrand factor antigen in Behçet's disease. *Clin Rheumatology* 1995; **14**(1): 55–61.

32. Cervera R, Navarro M, Lopez-Soto A et al. Antibodies to endothelial cells in Behçet's disease: cell-binding heterogeneity and association with clinical activity. *Ann Rheum Dis* 1994; **53**(4): 265–267.

33. Aydıntuğ AO, Tokgöz G, D'Cruz DP et al. Antibodies to endothelial cells in patients with BD. *Clin Immunol Immunopathol* 1993; **67**(2): 157–162.

34. Abdallah MA, Ragab N, Khalil R et al. Circulating immune complexes in various forms of BD. *Int J Dermatol* 1995; **34**(12): 841–845.

35. Knapp P. Beitrag zur Symptomatologie und Therapie der rezidiverenden Hypopyoniritis und der begleitenden apthösen Schleimhauterkrankungen. *Schweiz Med Wochenschr* 1941; **71**: 1288–1290.

36. Cavara V, D'Ermo E. A case of neuro-Behçet's syndrome. *XVII Concilium Ophthal Acta*, Canada, USA, 1954; **3**: 1489.

37. Al-Kawi MZ, Bohlega S, Banna M. MRI findings in neuro-Behçet's disease. *Neurology* 1991; **41**: 405–408.

38. Gürler A, Boyvat A, Türsen Ü. Clinical manifestations of Behçet's disease: an analysis of 2147 patients. *Yonsei Med J* 1997; **38**(6): 423–427.

39. Wechsler B, Vidailhet M, Piette JC et al. Cerebral venous sinus thrombosis in Behçet's disease: long term follow-up of 25 cases. *Neurology* 1992; **42**: 614–618.

disease and from HLA-B51 transgenic mice. *Arthr Rheum* 1995; **38**(3): 426–433.

40. Kansu T. Neuro-Behçet's disease. *Neurologist* 1998; **4**: 31–39.

41. Kansu T, Kansu E, Zileli T, Kırkali P. Neuro-ophthalmologic manifestations of Behçet's Disease. *Neuro-ophthalmology* 1991; **11**: 7–11.

42. Siva A, Özdoğan H, Yazici H et al. Headache, neuro-psychiatric and computerized tomography findings in Behçet's syndrome. In: Lehner T, Barnes CG, eds. *Recent Advances in Behçet's Disease.* London; RSM, 1986, 247–254.

43. Cengiz K, Özkan A. Psychiatric aspects of complete Behçet's syndrome: review of fifteen cases. In: O'Duffy JD, Kökmen E, eds. *Behçet's Disease: Basic and Clinical Aspects.* New York: Marcel Dekker, 1991, 115–118.

44. Perniciaro C, Molina J. Cerebrovascular aneurysms in patients with Behçet's disease. In: O'Duffy JD, Kökmen E, eds. *Behçet's Disease: Basic and Clinical Aspects.* New York: Marcel Dekker, 1991, 119–123.

45. Bussone G, La Mantia L, Boiardi A, Giovannini P. Chorea in Behçet's syndrome. *J Neurol* 1982; **227**: 89–92.

46. Bogdanova D, Milanov I, Georgiev D. Parkinsonian syndrome as a neurological manifestation of Behçet's disease. *Can J Neurol Sci* 1998; **25**(1): 82–85.

47. Pellechia MT, Cuomo T, Striano S et al. Paroxysmal dystonia in Behçet's disease. *Movement Dis* 1999; **14**: 177–178.

48. O'Duffy JD, Carney AJ, Deodhar S. Behçet's Disease, report of 10 cases, 3 with new manifestations. *Ann Intern Med* 1971; **75**: 561–570.

49. Baslo P, Kara I, Erek E et al. Clinical, electrophysiological, immunological and electron microscopic investigation of Behçet's disease. In: Dilşen N, Koniçe M, Ovul C, eds.

Behçet's Disease. International Congress Series 467. Amsterdam: Excerpta Medica, 1979, 178–182.

50. Namer IJ, Karabudak R, Zileli T et al. Peripheral nervous system involvement in Behçet's disease. *Eur Neurol* 1987; **26**: 235–240.

51. Takeuchi A, Kodama M, Takatsu M et al. Mononeuritis multiplex in incomplete Behçet's disease: a case report and the review of the literature. *Clin Rheumatol* 1989; **8**: 375–380.

52. Siva A, Necdet V, Yurdakul S et al. Neuroradiological findings in neuro-Behçet syndrome. In: O'Duffy JD, Kökmen E, eds. *Behçet's Disease: Basic and Clinical Aspects.* New York: Marcel Dekker, 1991, 323–329.

53. Banna M, El-Ramahi K. Neurological involvement in Behçet disease: imaging findings in 16 patients. *AJNR* 1991; **12**: 791–796.

54. Morrissey SP, Miller DH, Harmszewski R et al. Magnetic resonance imaging of the central nervous system in Behçet's disease. *Eur Neurol* 1993; **33**: 287–293.

55. Wechsler B, dell Isola B, Vidailhet M et al. MRI in 31 patients with Behçet's disease and neurological involvement: prospective study with clinical correlation. *J Neurol Neurosurg Psych* 1993; **56**: 793–798.

56. Koçer N, Işlak C, Siva A et al. CNS involvement in neuro-Behçet's syndrome: an MR study. *AJNR* 1999; **20**: 1015–1024.

57. McMenemey WH, Lawrence BJ. Encephalomyelopathy in Behçet's disease: report of necropsy findings in two cases. *Lancet* 1957; **24**: 353–358.

58. Kawakita H. Nishimura M, Satoh Y, Shibata N. Neurological aspects of Behçet's disease: a case report and clinico-pathological review of the literature in Japan. *J Neurol Sci* 1967; **5**: 417–438.

59. Totsuka S, Midorikawa T. Some clinical and pathological problems in neuro-Behçet's syndrome. *Folia Psychiatr Neurol Jpn* 1972; **26(4)**: 275–284.

60. Yamamori C, Ishino H, Inagaki T et al. Neurobehçet disease with demyelination and gliosis of the frontal white matter. *Clin Neuropathol* 1994; **13**: 208–215.

61. Hadsfield MG, Aydın F, Lippman HR, Sanders KM. Neurobehçet disease. *Clin Neuropathol* 1997; **16**: 55–60.

62. Serdaroğlu P, Yazıcı H, Özdemir C et al. Neurological involvement in Behçet's syndrome: a prospective study. *Arch Neurol* 1989; **46**: 265–269.

63. Akman-Demir G, Baykan-Kurt B, Serdaroğlu P et al. Seven-year follow-up of neurological involvement in Behçet's syndrome. *Arch Neurol* 1996; **53**: 691–694.

64. Kurtzke JF. Rating neurological impairment in MS: an expended disability status scale (EDSS). *Neurology* 1983; **33**: 1444–1452.

65. O'Duffy JD, Goldstein NP. Neurologic involvement in seven patients with Behçet's Disease. *Am J Med* 1976; **61**: 170–178.

66. Bang D. Treatment of Behçet's disease. *Yonsei Med J* 1997; **38(6)**: 401–410.

67. Hamuryudan V, Mat C, Saip S et al. Thalidomide in the treatment of the mucocutaneous lesions of the Behcet syndrome. A randomized, double-blind, placebo-controlled trial. *Ann Intern Med* 1998; **128(6)**: 443–450.

68. O'Duffy JD, Robertson DM, Goldstein NP. Chlorambucil in the treatment of uveitis and meningoencephalitis of Behçet's disease. *Am J Med* 1984; **76**: 75–84.

69. Kaveri SV, Mouthon L, Kazatchkine MD. Immunomodulating effects of intravenous immunoglobulin in autoimmune and inflammatory diseases. *J Neurol Neurosurg Psych* 1994; **57** (**suppl**): 6–8.
70. Van Schaik IN, Vermeulen M, Brand A. In vitro effects of polyvalent immunoglobulin for intravenous use. *J Neurol Neurosurg Psych* 1994; **57** (**suppl**): 15–17.
71. Dalakas MC. Mechanism of action of intravenous immunoglobulin and theraupetic considerations in the treatment of autoimmune neurologic diseases. *Neurology* 1998; **51** (**suppl 5**): S2–S8.
72. Lockwood CM. Intravenous immunoglobulin for the treatment of vasculitides. In: Kazatchkine MD, Morell A, eds. *Intravenous Immunoglobulin Research and Therapy*. New York: Parthenon, 1996, 143–145.
73. Boman S, Ballen JL, Seggev JS. Dramatic responses to intravenous immunoglobulin in vasculitis. *J Intern Med* 1995; **238**: 375–377.

10

West syndrome and Lennox–Gastaut syndrome

Willy O Renier

> CNS: central nervous system; CSF: cerebrospinal fluid; EEG: electroencephalogram; Ig: immunoglobulin; IVIG: intravenous immunoglobulin; LGS: Lennox–Gastaut syndrome; WS: West syndrome

Introduction

The central nervous system (CNS) has long been considered to be an immunologically isolated organ because the brain contains relatively few cells with the class II major histocompatibility complex molecules or antigen-presenting cells. Once a pathogen has penetrated the blood–brain barrier, the CNS was considered defenceless against the invader. In recent years this concept has changed. The CNS and the immune system are not independent networks. Far from being an immunologically privileged organ, the brain can regulate or shape immune responses, and immune responses can alter brain functions. The interactions between the immune and neuroendocrine systems have been the subject of rapidly expanding research. There is abundant receptor and ligand promiscuity.[1] The interactions between the nervous system and the immune system, however, have not yet been fully explained and the most fundamental questions concerning these interactions remain unsolved. One reason is that both complex systems are difficult to study in isolated conditions.

In the traditional concept, immunology might seem to have little to do with epilepsy, but scattered in the immunological, neurological and paediatric literature are several indications supportive of interactions between the immune system and the CNS in epilepsy (*Table 10.1*). Immunological factors may contribute to the development of epilepsy. It is possible that as a result of seizures, CNS antigens may become exposed to and trigger the immune system. Another possibility is misregulation of the immune system in epilepsy, due to a common genetically determined susceptibility or underlying biological process that during development concurrently gives rise to immune misregulation and to CNS disturbances leading to epilepsy.

The malignant epilepsies of childhood are a large group of epilepsies with a great diversity of clinical manifestations. They can be subdivided into age-related epileptic encephalopathies, a group characterized by alternating hemiconvulsions, and epilepsy with continuous spikes and waves during sleep. The first group is constituted by a spectrum of epilepsy syndromes: the neonatal or infantile epileptic encephalopathies with suppression bursts in the interictal electroencephalogram (EEG), the infantile spasms with hypsarrhythmia in the interictal EEG (West syndrome), and the Lennox–Gastaut syndrome with the slow spike and wave complexes in the interictal EEG.[2] They are called 'malignant epilepsies' because of developmental arrest or regression when seizures start. The seizures have to be considered as the clinical expression of an encephalopathic process. The epilepsy syndromes can be classified according to aetiology into idiopathic, cryptogenic and symptomatic. Idiopathic refers to a pure functional cerebral dysfunction, while cryptogenic and symptomatic refer to an encephalopathy with respectively unknown and known aetiology.[2]

Treatment of intractable epilepsies with immunoglobulins

The treatment of intractable epilepsies with immunoglobulins (Igs) started empirically. In 1977 Péchadre et al[3] reported that children with epilepsy who were treated with intramuscular injections of immunoglobulins (total Ig dose 0.66 g/kg) for recurrent infections of the upper respiratory tract experienced a decrease in the frequency and severity of their seizures. When

Table 10.1
Reported interactions between the immune system and CNS in epilepsies.

In humans
Reported immunogenetic abnormalities in patients with epilepsy:
  increased incidence of antibodies against brain tissue
  association with certain HLA alleles
  impaired immunity: IgG2 and IgA deficiencies; increased humoral or cellular immunity; lower kappa/lambda ratios of total Ig, IgG, IgM; decreased CD4/CD8 ratios; increased percentage of B cells
Effects of some antiepileptics:
  phenytoin and carbamazepine can suppress the immune system (lowering IgG2 and IgA) or precipitate systemic lupus erythematosus in some patients
  vigabatrin interferes with the cellular immune response
Immunosuppressive drugs, such as ACTH or corticosteroids, can show an anticonvulsant effect, especially in epilepsies of infancy such as West syndrome or Lennox–Gastaut syndrome
Clinical experience of exacerbation before and remission after infections of epilepsy in young children
Some immunologically mediated diseases such as systemic lupus erythematosus and myasthenia gravis are associated with epilepsy more often than would be expected by chance
Patients with gliomas and epilepsy present with suppression of humoral and cellular immunity
Rasmussen's encephalitis has been considered as an immunologically mediated cortical lesion with epilepsia partialis continua

In experimental animals
Epileptiform discharges can be recorded after intracerebral injection of antibrain antibodies to neuronal cell membrane components
Electroconvulsive shock induces production of antibrain antibodies
Antibrain autoantibodies from rats exposed to electroconvulsion show neuromodulating activity
Electrically and chemically induced convulsions modulate experimental allergic encephalomyelitis and other immune inflammatory reactions
Genetically epilepsy-prone rats show immune dysfunction (decreased IgM concentrations, increased IgG concentrations)
The immune response evokes changes in brain noradrenergic neurons

---

these researchers expanded their first results in 10 children to a group of 80, the success rate dropped from 90% to 65%.[4] Their observation revived the old allergic approach to epilepsies, and transformed it into an immunological one.

After 1977, a number of reports appeared

Table 10.2
Reported data on immunoglobulin treatment (MEDLINE, 1966–1993).

Number of studies	24
Number of patients	368
Age	<1–35 yr (mean 7.6 yr)
F/m ratio	1 : 2
Type of epilepsy	Various
idiopathic	124
WS	6 (4 WS, 2 WS + LGS)
LGS	4 (2 LGS, 2 WS + LGS)
IgG2 deficiency	49
Total dose Ig (g/kg)	0.3–6.8 (mean 2.4)
Duration (months)	0.15–12 (mean 4.0)
Efficacy:	
seizure reduction (%)	52 (0–90)
seizure freedom (%)	23 (0–80)
EEG improvement (%)	48 (0–90)
behaviour improvement (%)	72 (20–90)

on mostly successful intravenous immunoglobulin (IVIG) treatment in intractable epilepsies. Using MEDLINE, in the English, French and German literature from 1966 to 1993 there were 24 reports with a total of 368 patients. Only 6 cases of West syndrome (WS) and 4 cases of Lennox–Gastaut syndrome (LGS) were mentioned (*Table 10.2*). These uncontrolled clinical observations showed on the average a mean clinical seizure reduction and mean EEG improvement of 52% and 48%, respectively. On average, the percentage of patients with complete seizure remission and the percentage of patients with behavioural improvement were 23% and 72%, respectively. These studies suggest that IVIG may be effective in some patients with intractable epilepsy. However, cumulative metaanalysis of all identified articles is not possible because of the heterogeneity in study design, inclusion criteria, types of epilepsy, patient characteristics, treatment regimens, and method of evaluation of outcome. Nevertheless some tentative conclusions can be drawn from these studies. It does not matter at what age immunoglobulin therapy is started. Girls react better than boys. Idiopathic and cryptogenic types of epilepsy have better outcome than symptomatic types. IgG2 deficiency is not a prerequisite for a good outcome. High dosage of immunoglobulins per time unit is to be recommended. Adverse effects of IVIG as add-on medication are minimal.

With this knowledge in mind, a study was instituted in accordance with the Guidelines for Clinical Evaluation of Antiepileptic Drugs. This was a prospective add-on pilot study of high-dose IVIG administered to a homogeneous group of 15 children with cryptogenic WS and LGS. Conventional antiepileptic drugs, consisting of valproate and a benzodiazepine, mostly nitrazepam, were unchanged during the trial. The immunoglobulins were given intravenously in a quantity of 400 mg/kg body weight during 5 consecutive days and then the same dose was given once every 2 weeks for 3 months. Details of the study design are specified in the original article.[5] No clinical adverse effects were seen either during or after 165 infusions. The reduction in clinical seizure frequency averaged 70%, and mean reduction in epileptic discharges on EEG, blindly measured, was 40%. Psychomotor development after 3 months, measured by observation of behaviour and by the Denver developmental scale, improved in all patients. Observation revealed increased eye contact, attentiveness, perception and social adjustment. The amelioration of behaviour correlated with improvement of EEG background. The first clinical signs of improvement of the epileptic activity were noted 4–6 weeks after the start of treatment.

Behaviour and social contact improved sometimes even before seizure reduction. The latter observation has been mentioned by Péchadre et al.[4] This study in a well-defined group of patients with intractable epilepsy of infancy and young childhood provides additional arguments that IVIG should be considered when other treatments have failed.

Following IVIG administration, IgG concentrations increased in the serum in all patients, but also in the cerebrospinal fluid (CSF). All patients had an undisturbed blood–CSF barrier permeability before IVIG administration, as measured by Q albumin. CSF IgG increased in all patients except one.[5,6] The percentage of increase of CSF IgG was not associated with an equal percentage of increase of serum IgG. A higher amount of CSF IgG increase was not correlated with a faster or better seizure reduction. This study was the first to demonstrate that intravenously administered IgG molecules can reach the CNS.[6]

Indications of immunological dysfunction in West and Lennox–Gastaut syndromes

The most important intractable epilepsy syndromes in infancy and young childhood are WS and LGS. The LGS is an uncommon, unexplained age-related epileptic encephalopathy.[2] Various pathophysiologic mechanisms have been suggested to explain this condition, including the hypothesis that it results from aberrant or immature immune function. Indications supporting the hypothesis of a disturbed immune function include the demonstration of antibodies to brain tissue in the sera of patients with LGS, the effect of IVIG in young patients with LGS, and the indication of an impaired humoral immune response to a primary antigen (haemocyanin),[7] which has also been described in an autoimmune disease such as systemic lupus erythematosus. The total kappa/lambda ratios of total immunoglobulins, IgG and IgM are lower, while mean serum concentrations of total Ig, IgG and IgM are higher in epileptic children.[8] A low IgG2 is more frequent in very young children and has to be considered a physiological age-related phenomenon. It cannot be considered a prerequisite for a favourable response to IVIG. To investigate further the possibility that LGS of cryptogenic aetiology may be associated with autoimmune abnormalities, serologic HLA-A, B, C and especially HLA-DR and DQ typing studies were performed on 12 patients. A significant increase was found in the frequency of DR5 antigen and an indication of a decrease in the frequency of DR4 antigen as compared with a large group of normal control children. No significant differences in the frequencies of HLA-A, B and C antigens existed between the LGS group and the controls.[9]

Conclusion

Many clinical trials in malignant childhood epilepsies suffer from methodological shortcomings. A prospective clinical study by the author's department in a homogeneous group of children with a cryptogenic type of West or Lennox epilepsy has demonstrated that intravenous immunoglobulins can be effective in such cases. Additional studies support the hypothesis that immunogenetic mechanisms may play a part in triggering or maintaining intractable epilepsies in infants and children. Because many of the epilepsy syndromes in infancy and childhood are intractable, small results have value and all available methods of treatment should be fully exploited.

References

1. Van Engelen BGM. *A neuroimmunological approach of intractable childhood epilepsies.* Medical Thesis, University of Nijmegen, 1995.

2. Renier WO. The malignant epilepsies of childhood and adolescence. In: Aldenkamp AP, Dreifuss FE, Renier WO, Suurmeijer TPBM, eds. *Epilepsy in Children and Adolescents.* New York: CRC Press, 1995, 43–58.

3. Péchadre JC, Sauvezie B, Osier C, Gibert J. Traitement des encéphalopathies épileptiques de l'enfant par les gammaglobulines. *Rev EEG Neurophysiol* 1977; 7: 443–447.

4. Péchadre JC, de Villepin A, Sauvezie B,

Gibert J. Gamma-globulines et épilepsie. *Rev Méd* 1978; **34**: 1889–1901.

5. Van Engelen BGM, Renier WO, Weemaes CMR et al. High-dose intravenous immunoglobulin treatment in cryptogenic West and Lennox-Gastaut syndrome; an add-on study. *Eur J Pediatr* 1994; **153**: 762–769.

6. Van Engelen BGM, Renier WO, Weemaes CMR et al. Cerebrospinal fluid examinations in cryptogenic West and Lennox-Gastaut syndrome before and after intravenous immunoglobulin administration. *Epilepsy Res* 1994; **18**: 139–147.

7. Van Engelen BGM, Weemaes CMR, Renier WO et al. A dysbalanced immune system in cryptogenic Lennox-Gastaut syndrome. *Scand J Immunol* 1995; **41**: 209–213.

8. Haraldsson A, van Engelen BGM, Renier WO et al. Light chain ratios and concentrations of serum immunoglobulins in children with epilepsy. *Epilepsy Res* 1992; **13**: 255–260.

9. Van Engelen BGM, de Waal LP, Weemaes CMR, Renier WO. Serologic HLA typing in cryptogenic Lennox-Gastaut syndrome. *Epilepsy Res* 1994; **17**: 43–47.

11

Intravenous immunoglobulins: preparation, safety and clinical use

**Rainer H Böger and
Stefanie M Bode-Böger**

> AIDS: acquired immune deficiency syndrome; ALT: alanine transaminase; ANCA: antineutrophil cytoplasmic autoantibody; CIDP: chronic inflammatory demyelinating polyneuropathy; CJD: Creutzfeldt–Jakob disease; CMV: cytomegalovirus; EC: European Community; ELISA: enzyme-linked immunosorbent assay; EMA: European Medical Agency; Fab: fragment, antigen-binding; Fc: fragment, crystallizing; FDA: Food and Drug Administration; HBsAg: hepatitis B surface antigen; HBV/HCV: hepatitis B/C virus; HIV: human immunodeficiency virus; Ig: immunoglobulin; ITP: idiopathic thrombocytopenic purpura; IVIG: intravenous immunoglobulin; NIH: National Institues of Health; PCR: polymerase chain reaction; PEG: polyethylene glycol; WHO: World Health Organization

Introduction

Immunoglobulins—antibodies—are the most important effectors of the humoral defence reaction. Their therapeutic use has been possible since 1946 when Cohn first developed the ethanol fractionation of plasma (later known as Cohn fractionation).[1] Fraction II prepared according to this procedure contains plasma γ-globulins. After Bruton described a new disease characterized by the inability to produce circulating antibodies (Bruton agammaglobulinaemia),[2] prophylactic intramuscular injection of Cohn fraction II—termed immune globulin— became the treatment of choice for these patients. The intravenous administration route was avoided because of severe anaphylactic reactions which are due to massive complement activation by immunoglobulin aggregates. These are inevitably formed by the Cohn process.[3,4]

It has only been since modification of the immune globulin preparations that immunoglobulin G (IgG) may be given relatively safely by intravenous administration.[5,6] Because of this, immunoglobulin therapy has experienced a rapid expansion of its therapeutic uses from mere substitution therapy in patients with primary immunodeficiency to other therapeutic uses vaguely defined as 'immunomodulatory effects' of immunoglobulins.[7] Although intravenous immunoglobulins (IVIGs) have been tried in many diseases, a proven beneficial effect has only been seen in a few. Moreover, during recent years other problems have emerged: technical progress in the isolation of immunoglobulins from plasma has led to availability of numerous commercial products worldwide, which differ more or less obviously in some of their properties. Besides products that retain the physiological spectrum of antibody activity according to the population from which they were derived ('polyspecific immunoglobulins'), some preparations are available that are claimed to have enhanced activity against certain antigens ('specific immunoglobulins' or 'hyperimmunoglobulins'). Reports of viral infections caused by IVIGs have raised concerns about the viral safety of these products in recent years.[8,9] The rapidly expanding applications for IVIGs beyond labelled indications have led to concerns about the adequacy of many of these uses and—in the light of reduced health budgets—about the cost of this therapy.[10]

It is the purpose of this review to summarize the steps introduced into the preparation of IVIGs by different producers to meet the requirements of activity, antibody content, and safety of modern IVIG preparations. The variation in production steps between different manufacturers of commercially available IVIGs in Europe and the USA result in different pharmacological properties of the IVIG products (e.g. IgA content, addition of sugars and/or albumin, etc.), which may constitute criteria for the selection of a specific IVIG product in a specific patient or group of patients.

Comparing the pharmacological properties of IVIG products will help hospital drug committees find the IVIG product that best fits the specific need in a given patient population. This chapter briefly reviews the established and disputed clinical uses of IVIGs, and describes the ways in which the pharmacological properties may affect the selection of a product.

Structure and function of natural immunoglobulins

Immunoglobulins are mediators of the humoral immune response. They are produced by activated B cells upon contact with antigens. Five classes of immunoglobulins can be differentiated according to their biological properties: IgA, IgD, IgE, IgG and IgM. All immunoglobulins are composed of two heavy (H) chains and two light (L) chains, which are connected by intra- and intermolecular disulphide bonds (*Fig. 11.1*). Several molecular fragments can be distinguished according to the fragmentation behaviour of immunoglobulins during technical processing: the N terminal part of an H chain and one L chain form the Fab fragment; both Fab fragments are named F(ab)$_2$ fragment; the C terminal parts of both H chains form the Fc fragment of an immunoglobulin (*Fig. 11.1*). These fragments exert different functions within the immunoglobulin molecule: each Fab fragment contains an antigen binding domain which, because of the high variability of its amino

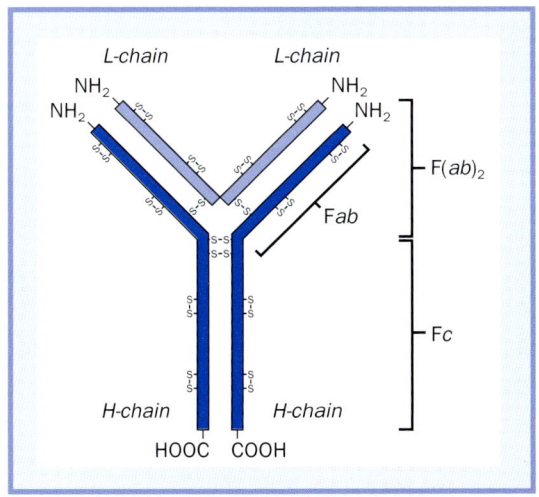

Figure 11.1
Structure of immunoglobulin G.

acid sequence, is responsible for the great diversity of antigens that can be recognized by different immunoglobulins. The F(ab)$_2$ fragment acts as a bivalent antibody; it can precipitate molecular antigens or agglutinate cellular antigens, and it can induce complement activation via the alternate pathway. The Fc fragment has no antigen binding ability, but it contains the characteristic properties of the different immunoglobulin classes, such as complement binding (IgG), placenta passage (IgG), tissue specificity and distribution in body fluids (e.g. secretion of IgA) and monocyte binding (IgE), and it determines the biological half-life of the immunoglobulins.

Immunoglobulin G comprises about 70% of total immunoglobulins in serum (*Table 11.1*). Its mean biological half-life is about 21 days, with major differences among the IgG subclasses: IgG1 (about 60% of total serum IgG), IgG2 (about 30%) and IgG4 (about 3%) have a mean half-life of 21 days, whereas IgG3 (about 7%) has a much shorter half-life of only about 7 days.[11] With its two antigen binding domains, IgG can precipitate molecular antigens or agglutinate cellular antigens;[12] antitoxins belong to the IgG class (IgG1), as do many antiviral (IgG1, IgG3) and antibacterial antibodies (IgG1, IgG2). The Fc fragment of IgG is responsible for complement activation via the classical pathway (mainly by IgG3), and for the binding of IgG4 to the surface of basophils and mast cells. IgG is equally distributed intra- and extravasally; it is the only immunoglobulin to pass the placental barrier in the third trimester of pregnancy and supply the newborn with maternal antibodies.

Immunoglobulin M makes up some 10% of total serum immunoglobulins. Its importance rises from the fact that IgM is the first antibody to be formed upon primary contact with an antigen (although IgM cannot pass the placental barrier, newborns can already synthesize their own IgM upon prenatal antigen exposure, e.g. to toxoplasmosis). IgM consists of a pentamer of five Ig monomers. It has the strongest ability for antigen lysis, agglutination and complement activation.

Immunoglobulin A makes up 15–20% of total immunoglobulins, of which only a small portion is present in serum.[13] Most IgA is secreted by exocrine glands; IgA is the main immunoglobulin in saliva, tears, and bronchial and intestinal fluids; it consists of an immunoglobulin dimer and a secretory polypeptide.

Immunoglobulin E is present in very low concentrations in serum of healthy humans, where it makes up less than 1% of total immunoglobulins. However, its synthesis is increased in allergic reactions and in immune reactions against parasitic infections; in these diseases elevated serum levels of IgE can be found.

Immunoglobulin D is also present in very

Table 11.1
Physiological characteristics and functions of natural immunoglobulins.

Immunoglobulin	Serum concentration (mg/dl)	Percentage of total body Ig	Physiological functions	Approximate half-life (days)
IgG	800–1800	70	Late antibody response against bacteria (IgG2, IgG1), viruses (IgG1, IgG3), and toxins (IgG3, IgG1); complement activation (IgG3, IgG1)	21
IgG1	c. 800	60		21
IgG2	c. 400	30		21
IgG3	c. 80	6		7
IgG4	c. 40	3		21
IgM	60–280	10	Early antibody response against bacteria, viruses	5
IgA	90–450	15–20	Secretory immunoglobulin on mucosal surfaces	6
IgE	0.001–0.014	≤1	Allergy, anaphylaxis, parasite infection, mast cell activation	2
IgD	0.3–40	≤1	Lymphocyte differentiation (?)	3

low concentrations in human serum (≤1%). It is an important antigen specific receptor on the lymphocyte surface; however, its biological function is not yet well characterized.

Requirements for intravenous immunoglobulins

An optimal commercially available immunoglobulin preparation should resemble the natural γ-globulins as closely as possible and retain as many as possible of their biological properties. As the different processes used in the fractionation of plasma and the processing of the IVIG preparation may cause modification of its biological properties, minimum requirements were first proposed by the World Health Organization[14] in 1982 (*Table 11.2*), and later defined by regulatory agencies such as the European Agency for the Evaluation of Medicinal Products for the European Union[15] or the Paul Ehrlich Institute for Blood and Blood Products in Germany.[16] The US Food and Drug Administration (FDA) has applied similar criteria, although these have not been explicitly published.

The distribution of antibody titres in IVIG preparations is not dramatically affected by the production process; instead it is influenced mainly by the source material, i.e. by the immunization status of the blood donor pool.[17] This confirms the observation of lot-to-lot variations in specific antibody titres among products from the same manufacturer,[18] and underscores three requirements for IVIG preparations:

(a) the need to combine plasma collected from a very large donor pool in order to minimize lot-to-lot variations in antibody titres;

(b) the testing of antibody titres against common antigens (e.g. hepatitis A virus, parvovirus B-19, cytomegalovirus) for each lot of the IVIG product;

(c) an optimal antibody spectrum according to the population to be treated (which is generally accomplished by using blood donors from the same population).

Production procedure

The basis for the preparation of all immunoglobulin preparations is the Cohn–Oncley fractionation of plasma.[1] A modification developed by Kistler and Nitschmann[19] is also widely employed in several European countries. These fractionation procedures involve the manipulation of pH, protein concentration, alcohol concentration, ionic strength and temperature, to selectively precipitate the various proteins of plasma. Other constituents of plasma such as coagulation factors and albumin are separated; fraction II generated by the cold ethanol fractionation consists of essentially pure IgG with only trace amounts

Table 11.2
Quality requirements for intravenous immunoglobulins.

Parameter	WHO	EMA	FDA
Size of donor pool	>1000	>1000	The FDA has not published any specific requirements on IVIG products to the best of the author's knowledge. However, requirements of the FDA closely resemble those of the EMA
Quality control	Transmit no infection	Transmit no infection At 5% protein (w/v) at least 3-fold concentration of Ab as compared to native plasma; at least 2 Ab activities (1 bacterial, 1 viral) controlled by international standards	
	Normal subclass distribution Intact Fc immunoglobulin function	Defined subclass distribution Intact Fc immunoglobulin function	
pH	NS	4.0–7.4	
Osmolality	NS	≥240 mosm/kg	
Protein content		≥3% (w/v) ± 10% of declared value	
	≥90% intact IgG As free as possible from aggregates	≥90% IgG mono- and dimers ≤3% polymers and aggregates	
Anticomplementary activity	NS	≤1 KH_{50}/mg IgG	
Prekallikrein activator	None	≤35 IE/ml at 3% (w/v) IgG	
Anti-AB haemagglutinins	NS	No haemagglutination at 1 : 64	
Pyrogens	None	None	
Anti-HBs antibodies	≥0.1 IU/ml	≥0.5 IU/g IgG	

Data from the WHO[14] and the European Pharmacopoea.[15] NS: not specified.

of other proteins such as IgA or IgM (*Fig. 11.2*). The maximal yield of IgG is about 5 grams per litre of plasma, while average commercial yields are about 2.5 g/l. Fraction II serves as the starting material for all IgG preparations, which are produced by removing residual alcohol from the precipitate by freeze-drying. Further steps are required to improve intravenous tolerance of immunoglobulins and to reduce the risk of viral transmission.

The production procedure may influence the distribution of IgG subclasses and the biological activities of the preparations as an indirect consequence of their sensitivity to enzymatic, chemical and/or physical treatment. This treatment is necessary to eliminate polymers and aggregates that are formed during the Cohn–Oncley fractionation of plasma. They comprise deliberate enzymatic cleavage (with plasmin or pepsin), chemical modification to split interchain disulphide bridges by reduction or alkylation, or to modify the Fc fragment (e.g. treatment with β-propiolactone, sulphonation), or chemical/physical treatment to remove aggregates from the product (e.g. pH 4 treatment, polyethylene glycol precipitation, adsorption, chromatography). In the production process of modern IVIGs, additional steps are included to reduce the probability of viral transmission (e.g. pasteurization, solvent/detergent treatment).

Pepsin or plasmin digestion was introduced early into the preparation of IVIGs because the aggregate formation of immunoglobulins and their complement activation depend on the activity of the Fc fragment, and both enzymes cleave the molecule between the Fc and Fab fragments. Plasmin cleaves the immunoglobulin molecule at a site above the disulphide bond linking the two heavy chains with each other (see *Fig. 11.1*). This results in the liberation of two free Fab fragments and one Fc fragment. The Fc fragments recovered in the preparation are no longer able to activate the classical complement cascade; however, they retain their binding capacity to Fc_γ receptors on different immune cells.[29] The IgG2 subclass of IgG is resistant to plasmin proteolysis; as a result, plasmin-treated IVIG preparations still contain a certain proportion of complete immunoglobulin molecules belonging to this subclass of IgG. These products are well tolerated because plasmin-treated Fc fragments have no anticomplementary activity, and because IgG2 is a weak activator of the complement system.[21]

Unlike plasmin, pepsin cleaves all four subclasses of IgG with equal efficacy at a site below the disulphide bond linking the two heavy chains (*Fig. 11.2*). This results in the liberation of one $F(ab)_2$ fragment and two remaining biologically inactive portions of the Fc fragment which are rapidly eliminated by

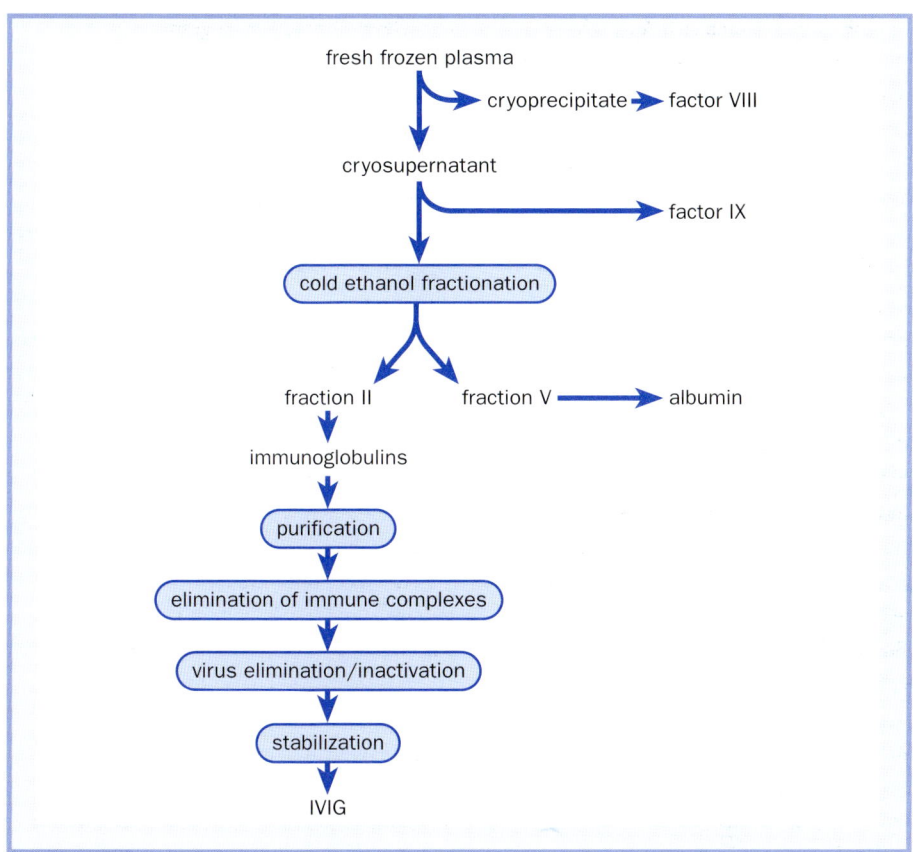

Figure 11.2
Production process of intravenous immunoglobulin preparations.

proteolysis or by renal excretion. Consequently, pepsin-treated immunoglobulin preparations are completely free of Fc fragments. The F(ab)$_2$ fragments migrate in the 5 S region during ultracentrifugation (corresponding to a molecular mass of about 100 kDa), whereas the complete immunoglobulin molecule migrates in the 7 S region (corresponding to a molecular mass of about 150 kDa). The 5 S immunoglobulins differ from 7 S immunoglobulin preparations in that their plasma half-life is reduced to about 36 hours, compared with about 20 days, and they lack the Fc-dependent functions of IgG (including the Fc-mediated suppression of the endogenous immune system).[22]

Several chemical modification procedures have been devised to counteract the autoaggregation tendency of IgG during the Cohn fractionation procedure while preserving the intact structure of the molecule. Chemical reduction of the IVIG preparation, followed either by alkylation/acetylation or by treatment with β-propiolactone, are procedures that introduce irreversible chemical modifications in the site of the Fc fragment responsible for aggregation. However, these chemical modifications potentially alter the physiological functions of the Fc fragments.[18]

The production of many modern immunoglobulin preparations involves one or more physical or chemical treatments which serve to eliminate aggregates while attempting to maintain the native structure and function of the molecule as well as preserving the physicochemical properties of the IgG subclasses and complete biological activity of the immunoglobulins. High-molecular-weight aggregates can be removed by additional fractional precipitation steps employing polyethylene glycol or ethanol, by ion exchange chromatography, by treatment with small quantities of pepsin at pH 4, or by incubating the product as a solution at pH 4 for 24 hours. In freeze-dried products, excipients such as human albumin, polyethylene glycol, glycine or sugars (sucrose, maltose, mannitol or glucose) may be added in order to minimize aggregation resulting from lyophilization, and to help maintain isotonicity (*Table 11.3*).[23]

Pharmacology

Immunoglobulin G is not absorbed to a significant extent following oral administration; after intramuscular administration time to peak plasma levels is about 5 days. After intravenous infusion, peak levels are attained within 30 minutes. Because of distribution of IVIGs between intra- and extravascular compartments, serum IgG levels drop by about 40–50% of the peak level during the first week following IV administration.[24] The half-life of elimination of IVIGs was determined to be approximately 24 days (2–3 weeks) in several investigations performed in neonates.[25–27] High concentrations of IVIGs and hypermetabolism associated with fever and infection may shorten the half-life of IgG.[24] The half-life of IVIGs is also reduced in bone marrow transplant recipients (30 hours to 10 days) compared with normal individuals,[28] but may be prolonged after long-term intravenous replacement therapy in adults with hypogammaglobulinaemia.[29]

Venous access for IVIG infusions every 2–3 weeks is a particular problem, especially for children with hypogammaglobulinaemias requiring regular and long-term substitution therapy. In these cases subcutaneous infusions have been tested as an alternate route of administration.[30] Infusions were reported to be well tolerated and effective.

Safety requirements

The transmission of infectious diseases is a major concern in the use of blood products. Since the WHO laid down minimum requirements for the preparation of immunoglobulins in 1982, evidence for immunoglobulin-associated transfer of non-A, non-B hepatitis (hepatitis C) in the mid-1980s has caused national and international authorities to issue stricter requirements for the safety of these products. Because of the need to include plasma from a large number of donations, there is an increased chance of viral transmission. Efforts to reduce the risk of transfection are directed by the following principles.

The best possible quality of the initial plasma

The guidelines issued by the EC in 1989 emphasize the importance of voluntary, unpaid blood donation.[31] Studies comparing paid donors with volunteer unpaid donors in the UK and in the USA have shown a higher prevalence of both HIV and HCV in commercial donors.[32,33] However, many manufacturers do not use plasma from first-time donors, and the rate of regular blood donors is much higher in commercial donor centres. With the introduction of good manufacturing practice standards, the quality of paid donor centres has improved in recent years. The majority of paid plasmapheresis centres are now located in low-risk areas, e.g. the midwestern part of the USA, and near university campuses. An additional step with regards to quality and safety can be taken by manufacturers by purchasing only plasma from donor centres that have been certified in the Quality Plasma Program. This certification, awarded by the American Blood Resources Association, exceeds FDA requirements.

Another point is related to Creutzfeldt–Jakob disease (CJD). Plasma taken from volunteer donations is usually recovered plasma from whole blood donations. Current thinking is that the risk of CJD contamination is higher in whole blood donations because of the presence of CJD in leukocytes. British plasma has recently been excluded from IVIG production for this concern.

Careful medical examination of every individual donor and appropriate questionnaires for anonymously eliminating any high-risk donors constitute further safeguards.

Table 11.3
Pharmacological, chemical and physical properties of commercially available IVIG products.

Preparation brand name	Manufacturer	Country of manufacture	Plasma pool N
Alphaglobin*† (Flebogamma IV-liquid pasteurized)	Instituto Grifols SA Barcelona, Spain	Spain	>1000
Biaven Iveegam (USA)	Farma-Biagini Lucca, Italy	Italy	NI
Endobulin*	Baxter/Immuno Vienna, Austria	Austria	>1000
Gammagard S/D	American Red Cross Washington DC, USA (Baxter/Hyland)	USA/Belgium	>1000
Gammar-P IV	Centeon Kankakee, IL, USA	USA	>1000
Gammonativ	Pharmacia & Upjohn Stockholm, Sweden	Sweden	6000–15 000
Intraglobin F*	Biotest Pharma Dreieich, Germany	Germany	1100–5000
Intrimun*	Biotest Pharma Dreieich, Germany	Denmark	1000–5000
Isivin	ISI Napoli, Italy	Italy	NI
Octagam*	Octapharma Vienna, Austria	Austria	>1000
Polyglobin 5%* Gamimune N (USA)	Bayer Leverkusen, Germany	USA	>2000
Sandoglobin*	Novartis Basel, Switzerland (Swiss Red Cross)	Switzerland	>16 000
Tégéline	LFB Les Ulis, France	France	NI
Venimmun N	Centeon Marburg, Germany	Germany	>1000
Venogamma	Finnish Red Cross Helsinki, Finland	Finland	6000–18 000
Venoglobin-S	Alpha Therapeutic Los Angeles, USA	USA	NI
Vigam-S	Bio Products Laboratory Elstree UK	UK	>1000
Vigam liquid§			

Plasma pool Origin	Preparation process	Additional steps for viral safety
USA Spain Czech Rep.	Cohn–Oncley PEG treatment	DEAE-Sephadex Pasteurization
NI	Cohn–Oncley Ion exchange	S/D
EU, USA	Cohn–Oncley PEG treatment	Nanofiltration
USA	Cohn–Oncley PEG treatment	DEAE Sephadex S/D, nanofiltration
USA	Cohn–Oncley	Pasteurization
Scandinavia	Cohn–Oncley Ion exchange	DEAE Sephadex S/D
Europe, USA	Cohn–Oncley	β-Propiolactone Nanofiltration
USA	Column chromatography PEG treatment Ion exchange	Pasteurization
NI	Cohn–Oncley	S/D pH 4 treatment
Austria, USA, Germany	Cohn–Oncley Column chromatography	S/D Viral neutralization pH 4 treatment
USA	Cohn–Oncley	S/D pH 4 treatment
Germany, Switzerland, USA	Kistler–Nitschmann Pepsin treatment	pH 4 treatment
Europe	Cohn–Oncley Pepsin treatment	pH 4 treatment Ultrafiltration
Germany	Cohn–Oncley Sulfitolysis	Nanofiltration
Finland	Cohn–Oncley Pepsin treatment	S/D Nanofiltration pH 4 treatment
USA	Cohn–Oncley PEG treatment	S/D pH 4 treatment
USA‡	Kistler–Nitschmann Ion exchange	S/D
		S/D pH 4 treatment

Table 11.3
Continued

Preparation brand name	IgG (% of total protein)	Monomers and dimers (%)	IgA content (µg/mol)
Alphaglobin*† (Flebogamma IV-liquid pasteurized)	≥97 [99.5]	≥93 [99.97]	<50 [9.5]
Biaven Iveegam (USA)	NI	NI	100
Endobulin*	≥99.9 [99.96]	≥90 [94.9]	≤55 [19.3]
Gammagard S/D	99	>90	<3
Gammar-P IV	>98	>90	<50
Gammonativ	NI	>96	8
Intraglobin F*	>95 [99.0]	>95 [98.8]	1500 [2090]
Intrimun*	>95 [100]	>99 [99.4]	<1
Isivin	99	100	118
Octagam*	>98 [100]	>90 [98.8]	≤100 [100]
Polyglobin 5%* Gamimune N (USA)	>98	100 [100]	<210
Sandoglobin*	>96	>90	<2400
Tégéline	[99]	[95.0]	[1080]
Venimmun N	≥97	NI	340
Venogamma	≥80	≥93	50
Venoglobin-S	>95	>90	<6
Vigam-S	>99	>94	<8
	99	≥98	<50
Vigam liquid§	100	99.4	

	IgG subclasses				Half-life (days)
IgG1 (%)	IgG2 (%)	IgG3 (%)	IgG4 (%)		
69 [67.8]	26 [28.4]	4 [2.0]	2 [1.8]		28 ± 8
NI	NI	NI	NI		24
50–80	20–50	<0.5	1–3		23–29
71	21	5	3		24
69	23	6	2		33.8
61	35	3	1		20–25
62	34	0.5	3.5		21.6
62	33	4	2		23.3
62–70	20–24	8.6–9.4	3.8–4.2		24
63	28.5	6.3	2.7		28
64.6	28.6	5.7	1.1		26.4
66	27	4.3	2.2		32
59	34	5	2		28 ± 9
63	27	3	7		21–36
62.4	33.6	3.4	0.3		NI
70	28	1.3	0.9		33.5 ± 7
56	38	5	1		28.9
		5.5	0.5		21

Table 11.3
Continued

	Sugars/stabilizers (g/l)	Albumin content (g/l)	Sodium content (g/l)	Osmolality (mosm/kg)
Alphaglobin*† (Flebogamma IV-liquid pasteurized)	D-sorbitol 50 [47.5] PEG ≤6 [4.56]	NA	NI	240–350 [313.4]
Biaven Iveegam (USA)	Sucrose?	NA	9	NI
Endobulin*	Glucose 45–55 [50.9]	NA	2–4 [3.0]	≥240 [390]
Gammagard S/D	Glycine 22.5 Glucose 20, PEG 2	3	9	NI
Gammar-P IV	Sucrose 4–6	2.4–3.6	5	NI
Gammonativ	Glucose? Glycine?	50	9	415
Intraglobin F*	Glucose 25 [25.7]	NA	1.8 [1.85]	≥240 [325.8]
Intrimun*	Sucrose 45	7.5	1.7 [1.85]	≥240 [302.6]
Isivin	Sucrose?	NA	8.5	450–600
Octagam*	Maltose 9–11 [10.5]	NA	≤7 [1.9]	≥240 [343]
Polyglobin 5%* Gamimune N (USA)	Maltose 10 [10]	NA	1.2	336 [342]
Sandoglobin*	Sucrose 102 ± 10 [99.7]	<1.8 [1.38]	3.6	>240 [433]
Tégéline	Saccharose 10	NI	0.8	375 ± 10
Venimmun N	Glycine?	NA	8.5	570–620
Venogamma	Sucrose 57–70	NI	1.0–1.3	380–460
Venoglobin-S	D-sorbitol 50 PEG ≤0.1	13	NI	300
Vigam-S	Sucrose 24 Glycine 3 Na-octanoate 0.6	20	2.3	340
Vigam liquid§				400

*Original data provided by manufacturer for proof. For these manufacturers, mean data from quality control certificates of at least five batches of the product are given in brackets. All manufacturers whose products are not marked by an asterisk failed to respond to repeated written requests for detailed product information. Abbreviations: NA: not applicable; NI: no information received or found; PEG: polyethylene glycol; S/D: solvent/detergent method of virus inactivation. For further details of product constituents and production/virus inactivation steps, see text.

Requirements for intravenous immunoglobulins 151

pH	Storage temperature	Maximum infusion rate (ml/min)	Form	Source of information
5.0–6.0 [5.66]	Room temp.	0.01–0.04 ml/kg·min	Liquid	Instituto Grifols Spain
c.6.8	Room temp.	NI	Powder	Turkish product brochure
6.4–7.2 [7.0]	Refrigerated	0.33	Powder	Immuno
6.8 ± 0.4	Room temp.	0.13 ml/kg·min	Powder	Intl English product brochure
6.4–7.2	Room temp.	0.06 ml/kg·min	Powder	English product brochure
6.7	Room temp.	3	Powder	Swedish Intl product brochure
6.8 [6.73]	Refrigerated	2	Liquid	Biotest Germany
6.6–6.9 [6.65]	Room temp.	3	Powder	Biotest Germany
7	Room temp.	NI	Powder	Turkish product brochure
5.1–6.0 [5.68]	Room temp.	3	Liquid	Octapharma Austria
4.0–4.5 [4.24]	Refrigerated	0.08 ml/kg·min	Liquid	Bayer Germany
6.4–6.8 [6.67]	Room temp.	2.5	Powder	Swiss Red Cross
NI	Refrigerated	0.07 ml/kg·min	Powder	French product brochure
6.4–7.2	Room temp.	2	Powder	German product brochure
6.0–7.0	Room temp.	NI	Liquid	Finnish Red Cross
5.2–5.8	Room temp.	0.08 ml/kg·min	Liquid	US product brochure
6.4–7.2	Room temp.	3	Powder	BPL
4.9	Refrigerated		Liquid	Product brochure

†Produced as Flebogamma for plasma of Spanish and Czech origin and marketed in these countries only; produced as Alphaglobin from US plasma for all other countries.
‡The plasma pool origin for Vigam-S has been changed to US plasma instead of British plasma because of theoretical concerns about the risk of a new variant of Creutzfeldt–Jakob disease in the UK blood supply, effective from November 1998.
§Only data for which this product differs from Vigam-S are separately listed in the table.

Individual donor screening

Individual screening of every blood or plasma donation should comprise tests for HBsAg, anti-HCV, anti-HIV-1 and -2, and syphilis serology. Normal values for alanine aminotransferase (ALT) are required in most countries. These test results must be unequivocally negative according to national donor guidelines, otherwise the blood or plasma donation must be rejected. Differences in the prevalence of these viruses have been published from different countries.[34–38] Quarantine storage of blood donations is another procedure allowing identification of potentially infectious samples if seroconversion of the donor occurs (and is detected) within the storage time of the blood donation. However, this applies only to regular blood donors, whereas late seroconversion will be missed in most irregular or single-occasion blood donors. Polymerase chain reaction (PCR) methods can be applied to detect minor amounts of some specific infectious viral DNA or RNA in plasma donations.

On the other hand, screening for antibodies will lead to IVIG preparations that lack certain antibodies because plasma donations which contain these antibodies are excluded from the production process (e.g. HCV, HIV). IVIGs therefore do not provide passive immunization against these diseases.

Virus inactivation procedures in the manufacturing process

It is now required by licensing authorities in Europe and the USA that at least one viral inactivation step be included into the manufacturing process of commercially marketed IVIG products. This measure has been introduced since the Cohn–Oncley ethanol fractionation itself has significant separation capacity for HIV and HBV,[39,40] but other viruses may still remain in the IgG fraction and cause infection of IVIG recipients. As an example, HCV RNA has been detected in immunoglobulins prepared according to the Cohn–Oncley procedure, despite the overall reduction in HCV load by a factor greater than 10^4.[41,42] Earlier IVIG preparations manufactured without a viral inactivation step were involved in the transmission of non-A, non-B hepatitis infection (later known as hepatitis C).[43–52] The safety of IVIGs with respect to viral transmission has recently been reviewed.[53]

Three methods of virus inactivation are used by manufacturers. The use of solvent/detergent is extremely effective against lipid-coated viruses such as hepatitis C, but has little activity against nonlipid-coated viruses such as parvovirus B-19. Pasteurization is employed by only a few manufacturers. It is effective against viruses sensitive to heat inactivation at 60 °C; however, this excludes many virus types. Further, the IgG molecule begins denaturation at 63 °C, thus requiring

Table 11.4
Test viruses used for the validation of virus inactivation and elimination procedures.

Actual virus tested	Model virus for	Virus group	Resistance to physicochemical treatment
Human immunodeficiency viruses 1 and 2	—	Enveloped, RNA, retroviruses	Low
Sindbis virus	HCV	Enveloped, RNA	Low
Pseudorabies virus	Herpesviruses	Enveloped, DNA	Medium
Vesicular stomatitis virus	Rhabdoviruses	Enveloped, RNA	Low
SV40 virus	Papovaviruses	Nonenveloped, DNA	Very high
Poliovirus	—	Nonenveloped, RNA	Medium
Animal parvoviruses	Parvoviruses	Nonenveloped, DNA	Very high
Parainfluenza virus	—	Enveloped, RNA	Low

extremely tight manufacturing controls. Betapropiolactone appears to be the most effective against both lipid-coated and nonlipid-coated viruses, but unfortunately it damages the Fc portion of the IgG molecule. Because no single primary method is totally effective, manufacturers employ additional secondary steps including incubation at pH 4, addition of pepsin, caprylic acid, polyethylene glycol and hydrolase treatment. Viral separation techniques are also employed by some manufacturers, including nanofiltration and column chromatography. Validation of these methods is still only partially standardized. Laboratories use model viruses because they are unable to grow enough of the actual viruses, e.g. hepatitis C virus (*Table 11.4*). There is no uniformity of model viruses among manufacturers, making it difficult to compare their data. Clinicians should require manufacturers to provide clear and understandable data with respect to viral safety and should consult a virologist for interpretation of ambiguous information.

The virus reduction factor is defined as the log_{10} of the ratio of the virus load in the prepurification material (i.e. source plasma) divided by the virus load in the postpurification material (i.e. the IVIG preparation). The manufacturing process as a whole is required to contain two independent steps allowing for a reduction of enveloped viruses by at least 4 log units each (total reduction of enveloped viruses by at least 10 log units), and one step reducing the load of nonenveloped viruses by 4 log units (total reduction of nonenveloped viruses by at least 6 log units). Companies are required to verify the efficacy of the viral inactivation procedures using plasma samples spiked with high loads of the virus or using model viruses.[54] Experimental studies showing the efficiency of different virus inactivation procedures have since been published for polyethylene glycol (PEG) treatment,[55,56] low pH treatment combined with pepsin,[57,58] solvent/detergent treatment,[59] β-propiolactone treatment[60] and others.[61] The solvent/detergent method is usually performed using tri-(n-butyl)phosphate as solvent and sodium cholate, Tween 80 or Triton-X as detergent. It can be inserted readily into any purification scheme, providing predictable and efficacious virus inactivation for coated viruses without affecting normal Fc functional activity.[62] Nonenveloped viruses will not be inactivated with this method; thus, protection against these viruses needs to come from other factors.[61] Alkylating substances like β-propiolactone are suitable for the inactivation of enveloped viruses, and of nonenveloped viruses to a lesser extent.[63] However, this method has not been widely adopted because β-propiolactone alkylates protein and may act as a carcinogen, although there is evidence that unreacted β-propiolactone hydrolyzes completely in plasma to noncarcinogenic β-hydroxypropionic acid.[61]

Although each of these methods seems to be effective, none can guarantee the total absence of infectious viruses. Although small clinical studies indicated the viral safety of IVIGs prepared by various methods,[64] for statistical reasons related to the small number of cases these studies cannot exclude the occurrence of infections by these preparations in the future.[65] Moreover, no process can guarantee effectiveness against viruses or other infectious particles still unknown. Known effective methods for the reduction of viral load always have an effect on the biological activity of the product, so that a balance between preservation of biological activity and compatibility and viral safety needs to be achieved. Therefore, it must be remembered that each immunoglobulin preparation is the product of a different manufacturing process so that products are not interchangeable. Indiscriminate use of more than one product in a given patient will prevent identification of the source of hepatitis C or other transmissible agent if such an infection occurs.[66] The potential risks of IVIG therapy must be considered before therapy is begun, particularly in diseases in which the benefits of treatment are not clearly established.[67] Recording the lot number and the manufacturer of the IVIG product in the patient's records allows identification of potentially infectious batches in case an infection should occur.

Other side-effects

Adverse reactions to immunoglobulins may be acute reactions occurring during or immediately after the infusion of the immunoglobulin, or delayed reactions which occur several hours, days or even longer afterwards. Acute reactions are mostly allergic in nature; they are the most frequent adverse events and may include symptoms ranging from a rash to severe anaphylaxis. Since mild allergic reactions are common and anaphylaxis cannot be predicted—it may even occur in patients never before treated with immunoglobulins—the first few intravenous infusions should be given very slowly, with antihistamine and hydrocortisone available. Adrenaline should always be available, even at home, in case of anaphylaxis. Anaphylaxis has been reported to be more common in patients who are IgA deficient and may have developed anti-IgA antibodies;[68] however, anaphylaxis may also be due to the immediate formation of immune complexes in patients without IgA deficiency.[68] The incidence of anti-IgA antibodies of various types may be as high as 18% in patients with hypogammaglobulinaemia.[69] IgA-free material should be used for patients with very high or rising titres of anti-IgA antibodies,[70] and patients with immunodeficiencies should be screened for the presence of IgA deficiency before receiving IVIGs. Anaphylactoid reactions have been attributed to the presence of IgG aggregates,[71] trace amounts of pepsin, sucrose, or β-lipoproteins.[7,68]

Other adverse reactions may be mild, moderate, or severe.[72] They may comprise acute reactions such as fever, chills and headache, which have been reported to occur in 2–6% of patients. Other reactions include abdominal cramps, nausea, emesis, muscle pain, anxiety, chest tightness and dizziness.[73] These adverse reactions are often related to the speed of infusion. Different products have different rates of infusion because of differences in stabilizers, total protein content, pH and particle count. It is important that persons actually administering the IVIG read the manufacturer's package leaflet for the rate of infusion recommended for that specific product. Reactions usually occur within the first hour of infusion. Should any of these reactions occur, stop the infusion, wait for 30 minutes, and restart at a slower infusion speed. Even with the recommended infusion rate, a large interpatient variability exists such that some patients tolerate a much faster infusion, while others require an even slower infusion speed. Some patients may react even with very slow infusion speed and to different brands. These rare patients may require prophylactic treatment 30 minutes prior to IVIG infusion with 50–100 mg hydrocortisone, an antipyretic, and/or an antihistamine.[74,75]

Local reactions that occur at the site of infusion include erythema, pain, phlebitis and eczematous reactions. Intravenous products with low pH at the time of infusion may produce systemic effects in patients with disturbed acid–base balance[73] and in neonates, as well as severe irritation and/or necrosis at the infusion site. Rare, less well-defined reactions may be erythema multiforme,[76] aseptic meningitis,[77,78] thrombotic events[79,80] (in one case stroke has been reported[81]), or haemolysis due to anti-AB haemagglutinins or anti-D antibodies.[82,83] Aseptic meningitis has been reported in up to 11% of neurologic patients receiving IVIGs.[78] It may mimic bacterial meningitis with neutrophilic pleocytosis, elevated protein concentration, and decreased glucose in cerebrospinal fluid. Normal treatment is symptomatic with narcotic analgesics and antiemetics.

Intravenous immunoglobulin will diminish the active immunity of measles vaccine, mumps vaccine, or rubella vaccine.[84,85] Patients receiving immunization concomitantly with IVIG therapy may lack seroconversion against the vaccine; they should be considered as candidates for revaccination after the end of IVIG therapy. Generally, it is recommended that the vaccine should be given 14 days before or 3 months after IVIG therapy.

Some adverse reactions can be attributed to constituents other than the immunoglobulins contained in commercially available products. Contamination of IVIGs with vasoactive enzymes such as prekallikrein activator or kallikrein has also been suggested as a possible mechanism for adverse reactions.[86] Osmotic nephrosis has been suggested to have been caused by the high concentration of sucrose in some products,[87] but a transient rise in serum creatinine concentration has been reported with various preparations which may be due to a tubular defect induced by IVIGs.[88] Patients with preexisting renal disease may be more prone to renal side-effects, and some authors recommend deferring the use of IVIG in patients with clinical evidence of rapidly progressive renal disease, as demonstrated by a 30% rise in serum creatinine levels in the preceding 2 weeks.[72] In addition, patients should be well hydrated, and concomitant diuretic use should be avoided, particularly in patients with preexisting renal disease.[87] Another consideration is that high sodium content in some preparations and the infusion of large volumes can cause fluid overload and congestive heart failure in predisposed patients.[89]

Comparison of commercially available IVIG preparations

Among commercially marketed IVIG preparations currently available in Europe and the USA some differences in preparation process, method of virus inactivation, and stabilization can be observed that may affect the choice of a specific preparation for a specific group of patients. Moreover, differences in the disease spectrum between different hospitals may cause drug committees to apply different priorities in brand selection.

This decision should, however, be based on objective pharmacologic criteria. A number of parameters may affect the choice of a specific IVIG product or its dosage, such as osmolality or IgA content. Underlying medical conditions that are not readily obvious in a given patient may also affect the choice of IVIGs; e.g. borderline renal failure may become relevant if during the administration of IVIGs serum creatinine levels rise.

Table 11.3 lists the main characteristics of IVIG preparations available in Europe and the USA. While the list is not intended to be complete, it comprises some of the main criteria which may be of importance for hospital drug committees in formulary selection.

While many IVIGs are produced in one country, some are produced in various countries and marketed under the same or under different brand names. Most IVIGs are marketed not only in their country of origin but also throughout Europe, and many are also available worldwide. The preparation process follows the original Cohn–Oncley procedure or its modification by Kistler and Nitschmann[19] for all products, but additional steps introduced for viral inactivation may vary. As more information becomes available on the viral safety of different procedures, it is important to be aware of the procedure by which a specific preparation is produced. The larger the pool of plasma donors for a given product is, the more stable will the antibody titres be. High purity of IgG and a high fraction of IgG present in the form of monomers and dimers are required by regulatory authorities today; these criteria are met by all manufacturers. The relative distribution of monomers and dimers may vary among products because of differences in pH. The content in IgA may be critical in groups of patients with a high prevalence of anti-IgA antibodies; in other patients this may be of less relevance. IgG subclass distribution should resemble as closely as possible the natural distribution of these subclasses; it is affected to different degrees by the various production processes. The half-life of the preparations may also vary according to the production process applied; however, differences among 7 S immunoglobulins listed here are much smaller in comparison to 5 S immunoglobulins. The addition of sugars and stabilizers as well as the content of albumin and sodium and the osmolality vary considerably between products. As these additives may be the source of side-effects in subgroups of patients, products should be selected accordingly. The pH of the final infusion may also affect patient outcome, at least when high doses are administered. Storage temperature is important logistic information for the pharmacist, as is the maximal infusion rate for the therapist.

Although antibody titres for some major antigens may vary considerably between products as well as between lots of a given product, this information is difficult to interpret. Reference standards for most antigens are lacking, so that antibody titres obtained in different laboratories may not be comparable; moreover, even for those antigens for which there are reference standards, antibody titres obtained by methods such as ELISA may not represent the true neutralizing potential of the product, as the tests may detect antigen moieties other than those required for infectiosity of the pathogens. Antigen neutralization assays have also not been standardized, so that even this information would not be of any comparative value. There are many studies comparing chemical, physical or pharmaceutical properties of IVIG products, but no study is available showing superiority with respect to clinical outcome of product over another in direct comparison.

In *Table 11.3* the source of information for each product is indicated; this is written information mailed from the manufacturer for most products. However, some manufacturers did not respond to repeated requests for information on their products; in these cases the information is obtained from marketing brochures. Moreover, many manufacturers provided copies of analysis certificates from several lots out of their current production. Products for which original data have been made available for review by manufacturers are marked by an asterisk; mean values from at least four different lots are given in brackets for these products.

Mechanisms of action

The mechanism of action of IVIGs is evident for patients with antibody deficiencies. In primary and secondary humoral immunodeficiencies IVIGs replace the natural immunoglobulins that are not formed in the body for various reasons, in order to maintain the natural function of the humoral immune system.

However, IVIG also has immunomodulatory actions which are not yet fully understood. In some situations, such as acquired factor VIII deficiency (which is due to endogenous anti-factor VIII antibodies), the capacity of IVIGs to block autoimmune reactions is clearly due to the presence of antiidiotypes which inhibit the pathogenic autoantibodies.[90,91] Less specified (and less understood) reactions may include the blockade or downregulation of Fc receptors, by which mechanism clearance and removal of opsonized cells cannot be accomplished,[92–94] the induction of suppressor cells,[95] the downregulation of complement activation which has been established in vitro[96] and in a guinea-pig model in vivo,[97] the presence of antibodies to cytokines,[98,99] the inhibition of endogenous immunoglobulin formation by IVIG,[100,101] or the downregulation of the immune system and inflammation by as yet undefined mechanisms.[102] Other characteristics of IVIGs may contribute to their immunomodulatory effects in some diseases. In particular, IVIGs show specific diffusion into the site of inflammation.[103] The presence of IgG dimers consisting of idiotype–antiidiotype complexes has also been suggested to influence the therapeutic effects of IVIGs.[23,104]

The understanding of these complex interactions of IVIGs with the immune system is relevant to our knowledge of its therapeutic effects in B-cell and in T-cell-mediated immunological diseases.[105]

Clinical uses

Currently IVIG is used for a myriad of different indications, of which only some are unequivocally proved and approved by regulatory authorities; in others IVIG use is supported by data from controlled clinical trials but not yet finally proved, and should therefore be considered a reserve therapy when other treatments have failed; in many other conditions IVIG use should be considered experimental because it is only supported by anecdotal reports or by theoretical considerations. The vast field of potential indications for which IVIGs have been tested and are currently being tested can therefore be subdivided into approved indications, probably (and possibly) effective indications, and experimental indications. Others have subdivided potential indications for IVIG into primary and secondary antibody deficiencies, treatment of specific infections, treatment of autoimmune diseases, and other inflammatory conditions. These categories of indications are used here to group various diseases in which the levels of evidence are similar.

Numerous reviews of the clinical uses of IVIGs have been published in recent years, some of which are excellent. These reviews are referred to where appropriate.

Approved indications

All IVIG products currently on the market have been proved to be effective and licensed for the treatment of primary antibody deficiency. Manufacturers are aware that because in this group of diseases antibody deficiency is the single pathogenetic cause it is readily responsive to IVIG substitution, and effectiveness can therefore be shown in clinical trials involving a relatively small number of patients.

Primary immunodeficiencies

Primary antibody deficiency has been the first clinical indication treated with intramuscular immunoglobulins. It has been recognized that primary antibody deficiencies are group of primary (inborn or acquired) immunological diseases which are due to various genetic defects (*Table 11.5*). With the exception of selective IgA deficiency, which occurs in about 1 per 700 population, these diseases are relatively rare. However, many patients are

Table 11.5
Primary antibody deficiencies and combined (B-cell and T-cell) immunodeficiencies in which IVIG treatment is indicated.

Diagnosis
Antibody deficiencies Common variable immunodeficiency X-linked antibody deficiency IgG subclass deficiencies in patients with recurrent infections Specific antibody deficiency with normal immunoglobulin levels Selective IgA deficiency in patients with deficient antibody production and recurrent infections **Combined immunodeficiencies** Severe combined immunodeficiency Wiskott–Aldrich syndrome Ataxia-telangiectasia X-linked lymphoproliferative syndrome **Low-birthweight neonates**

diagnosed late, which may in part be due to the common misconception that all primary immunodeficiencies present in childhood.[106] As an example, the great majority of patients with common variable immunodeficiency present after the age of 6 years, and many patients are first diagnosed in adolescence.[107] Untreated patients with unrecognized primary antibody deficiencies suffer from recurrent infections, some of which may be severe like pneumonia or meningitis,[107,108] and many will experience long-term complications such as failure to thrive, enteropathy, bronchiectasis and anaemia.[109,110]

The primary therapeutic goal of immunoglobulin replacement therapy in primary antibody deficiency is not to maintain a certain IgG plasma level, but rather is oriented at clinical criteria. The aims are to prevent further acute infections of the patient and to halt the progress of complications if present, but at the same time avoid the complications of replacement immunoglobulin therapy. However, one problem in assessing treatment efficacy is that reduction in occurrence of infections and complications in a given patient can only be assessed retrospectively; therefore, serum IgG levels serve as surrogate end-points although they do not necessarily correlate with clinical efficacy.

The efficacy of immunoglobulin

replacement therapy was first shown for intramuscular immunoglobulin in the British Medical Research Council trial in 1969.[111] However, for ethical reasons no placebo control group was included in this study; thus, there has never been a placebo-controlled study of the use of immunoglobulin replacement therapy in antibody deficiency diseases.[67] Intravenous immunoglobulins have since become the preferred treatment because higher IgG levels can be reached.[66,112] Roifman et al[113] demonstrated that infections occurred less frequently when serum IgG levels were above 5 g/l than when they were below 5 g/l during IVIG replacement therapy. Clinical studies support the benefits of IVIG treatment over intramuscular IgG.[107,112,114,115] High-dose IVIG has been shown to be superior to low-dose IVIG therapy.[113,116] Early IVIG regimens used 100–200 mg/kg per month, a dose sufficient to keep many patients symptom-free. Today most patients receive about 400 mg/kg per month, usually in two doses 2 weeks apart, as the half-life of the preparations is about 3 weeks; only very few patients require doses of up to 1 g/kg per month in divided doses.[66]

Deficiency of IgG subclasses is associated with an increased incidence of infection;[117,118] specifically, IgG$_2$ deficiency was linked with recurrent sinopulmonary infections[119,120] and poor antibody response to carbohydrate antigens in children.[121] However, although IgG subclass deficiency may be a marker of immune dysfunction and increase the likelihood that there will be a defect in antibody production, more refined studies have revealed that it is the inability to produce specific antibodies that is relevant to the susceptibility to infection.[120,122] IVIG substitution can reduce the incidence of infection and be beneficial in patients with an inadequate response to treatment with antibiotics.[123]

Selective IgA deficiency is considered a contraindication to the use of IVIGs, as most of these patients produce antibodies normally and IVIGs cannot replace antibodies at the mucosal surface.[67] Moreover, patients with selective IgA deficiency are at an increased risk of developing anaphylactic reactions to IVIG due to the presence of anti-IgA antibodies in their serum, and the presence of IgA in nearly all IVIG preparations (see *Table 11.3*). However, in a subgroup of these patients there is a defect in antibody production and these patients often suffer from recurrent infections. In this subgroup IVIG therapy may reduce the frequency of infections,[124,125] but the potential benefits of IVIGs must be weighed against the risk of serious or even life-threatening anaphylactic reactions.

Although there are no controlled studies for the use of IVIGs in combined immunodeficiencies, patients with defective antibody production may be treated with IVIGs even when the primary abnormality is absent T-cell function.[126–128] However, it should be remembered that IVIG replacement may reduce the incidence of bacterial and viral infections, but it will not affect the underlying defect or the incidence of malignancy.[67]

Low-birthweight neonates are at high risk of developing severe systemic bacterial infections which are most frequently caused by *Escherichia coli* or group B streptococci.[129] Antibody concentrations against these pathogens contained in different IVIG preparations may vary greatly, which may explain in part the controversial results obtained by different studies. Several studies showed beneficial results of IVIG treatment in neonatal sepsis,[130–133] but others yielded no benefit from IVIG treatment,[27] or showed short-term benefit but no long-term improvement of prognosis.[25] In summary, IVIG should not be used routinely in all neonates to prevent sepsis, but it may be appropriate for the prophylaxis of bacterial infections in preterm infants at high risk of sepsis.

Secondary immunodeficiencies

Secondary immunodeficiencies may be secondary to other diseases that affect the production of B cells in the bone marrow (leukaemias, bone marrow metastasis, paraneoplastic syndromes), that reduce the ability of B cells to produce functionally intact antibodies (acquired immunodeficiency syndrome), or that result in a disproportionate loss of protein including antibodies (burns, enteropathy, nephrotic syndrome). With increasing frequency, secondary immunodeficiencies are iatrogenic, occurring in patients whose immune system is artificially suppressed during chemotherapy, or in bone marrow transplant or solid organ transplant recipients who undergo immunosuppressive therapy. The major goal in these patients is to prevent infection, but the important infectious agents vary considerably, requiring that the clinical efficacy of IVIGs be established separately for each of these conditions.

Solid organ transplantation One major problem of patients after organ transplantation is cytomegalovirus (CMV) infection, which contributes considerably to the overall mortality of these patients.[134] The virus may be transmitted either by cellular blood products or by the donor organ.[135] Infection is facilitated by the severe immunosuppressive therapy that these patients need to undergo to prevent graft rejection. In seropositive patients reinfection with a second viral strain or reactivation of endogenous latent virus may occur. While CMV infection is asymptomatic in many immunocompetent patients, symptomatic CMV infection is more common in transplant recipients; it may develop in up to 80% of the transplant population.[136] Symptomatic CMV infection is often manifested as fever, malaise and leukopenia, but symptoms may include interstitial pneumonia, hepatitis, renitis and multisystem disease. The infected patient is at increased risk of bacterial, fungal and parasitic superinfection; impaired graft function and rejection may occur. Thus, CMV infection presents a significant threat to graft and patient survival in transplant recipients. Prophylaxis of CMV infection with IVIGs has been studied in a limited number of controlled clinical trials and in numerous uncontrolled trials.[137,138] IVIGs are therefore recommended in high-risk transplantation (seronegative recipient, seropositive organ). While this is established in renal and heart transplantation, the issue is more complex in heart–lung transplantation and in liver and pancreas transplantation, because in the former small patient numbers have prevented controlled clinical trials, and in the latter another risk is that of acute hepatitis B infection due to the high rate of HBV-positive organ recipients.[139,140]

IVIG treatment is only one measure besides the use of antibacterial, antiviral and antifungal antibiotics,[141,142] the use of haematopoietic growth factors to reduce the duration of neutropenia, and the use of CMV-free blood products to reduce the risk of infection. The risk–benefit ratio and the cost-effectiveness of these measures have not yet been studied comparatively.

Allogeneic bone marrow transplantation In patients after bone marrow transplantation CMV infection also contributes considerably to the overall morbidity and mortality.[143,144] IVIGs have been shown to protect bone marrow transplant recipients both from de novo infection as well as from reactivation of persistent virus.[145,146] Combination therapy with antiviral chemotherapy and IVIGs has now been shown to improve survival if started early in the course of the disease.[147]

In bone marrow transplant recipients, IVIGs may exert additional benefits by reducing the severity of graft-versus-host disease, although this has not yet been conclusively shown.[148–150] A more recent study showed that in the absence of hypogammaglobulinaemia, monthly administration of IVIGs does not reduce late complications and may impair long-term humoral immune recovery after bone marrow transplantation.[151]

Children with acquired immunodeficiency syndrome Paediatric AIDS patients have an increased susceptibility to bacterial and viral infections. In a large, randomized, placebo-controlled, multicentre trial including 372 children with AIDS children with CD4 lymphocyte counts above 200 cells/µl IVIG provided particular benefit for the prevention of infections as compared with placebo, whereas more severely ill children with CD4 lymphocyte counts below 200 cells/µl did not profit from this treatment.[152] Total mortality was similar in both groups. However, in this trial few children were treated with antiviral agents and few received prophylaxis for *Pneumocystis carinii* pneumonia; both measures would be standard treatment today. Future trials of IVIG in children who receive this additional therapy will help to clarify the role of IVIG in paediatric AIDS therapy.

Immunomodulatory effects of immunoglobulins

It was on grounds of anecdotal observation rather than theoretical considerations that immunoglobulins were applied for reasons other than providing antibodies. The observation that a hypogammaglobulinaemic, thrombocytopenic child showed an increase of his thrombocytes after IVIG infusion[153] started a new era of applying IVIGs for immunomodulatory treatment in different forms of autoimmune and immune complex diseases. Although IVIGs have been tried in many autoimmune diseases since then, a beneficial effect has only been proved in controlled clinical trials in a few. Moreover, even in some of those conditions in which a clinical benefit has been demonstrated in controlled trials, the mode of action has yet to be elucidated.

Idiopathic thrombocytopenic purpura
Idiopathic thrombocytopenic purpura (ITP) is caused by autoantibodies directed against platelet antigen. Binding of antibodies to the platelet surface accelerates phagocytosis of the platelets in the reticuloendothelial system.[154] The antiplatelet antibody is IgG in most cases; antiplatelet IgM and IgA have also been detected in serum of patients with ITP. Treatment of acute chronic ITP with IVIGs allows a rapid recovery in terms of higher thrombocyte counts and diminished bleeding in the great majority of cases. IVIGs seem to be especially effective in patients who are resistant to steroid treatment. The usual dose is 400 mg/kg per day for 5 consecutive days.[153,155]

Kawasaki's disease Kawasaki's disease (mucocutaneous lymph node syndrome) is an acute, febrile, exanthematous disease which was first reported in Japan in 1967.[156] The major complication of this disease is a cardiovacular manifestation leading to coronary aneurysms and thrombotic occlusion; this is associated with a high short-term and long-term morbidity and mortality.[157] Therapy aimed at reducing the incidence of coronary artery abnormalities was only available in the form of aspirin before the advent of IVIG treatment. IVIG administration has been shown to be effective in preventing coronary artery manifestation in this disease when IVIG treatment is started at an early stage (within 10 days after the onset of the disease).[145] The usual recommended dose is 400 mg/kg per day for 4 consecutive days.[145,146,158] Newburger et al reported the effectiveness of a single dose of 2 g/kg given over 10 hours;[159] this dosage has been adopted by an NIH Consensus Conference report.[145]

Guillain–Barré syndrome In patients with Guillain–Barré syndrome IVIG treatment may constitute an alternative to plasma exchange therapy.[160] Two major randomized, controlled studies comparing both therapeutic strategies have found that IVIG therapy is at least as effective as plasma exchange and better than no treatment.[161,162] IVIGs may be especially useful in patients in whom other therapy has failed or is contraindicated, or in whom venous access for plasma exchange is difficult.[163]

Probably or possibly effective indications

This group of indications comprises diseases in which IVIG treatment has been shown in controlled clinical trials to be effective, and which may be expected to be approved in the future. In other diseases an overall tendency of IVIG to be efficacious can be identified from clinical trials, but significant numbers of patients are unresponsive to IVIG treatment ('possibly effective' indications). It must be a subject of future clinical studies to improve the criteria by which 'IVIG responders' may be differentiated from 'IVIG nonresponders' before initiating treatment. Diagnostic criteria are needed to define the response to IVIG treatment (the therapeutic goal) in an individual patient, with the option to discontinue treatment in case of nonresponsiveness. Weighing the potential benefits of IVIG against its potential risks in comparison to the risk–benefit ratio of alternative treatments is of utmost importance in these diseases.

Secondary immunodeficiencies

Malignancies and chemotherapy Antibody deficiency is common in patients with chronic lymphocytic leukaemia, multiple myeloma and other cancers, especially in advanced stages of the disease and/or secondary to cytostatic therapy. IVIG treatment has been shown to reduce the incidence of major bacterial infections in patients with chronic lymphocytic leukaemia.[164] The number of trivial infections was unchanged. Other studies have shown that IVIG can reduce the frequency of infection in patients with multiple myeloma and with cancer of the lung.[165,166] However, as the cost-effectiveness of such treatment has not yet been established,[167] IVIG treatment is not widely recommended in these diseases, but it remains an option for patients at high risk of recurrent infections.[145,155,168]

Adult HIV infection and AIDS The use of IVIG in HIV-infected adult patients has not been studied in many well-controlled trials. In contrast to children with AIDS, infections with common bacteria are less frequent in adult AIDS patients. One controlled trial has shown that adult patients with advanced AIDS had fewer serious infections during IVIG treatment compared with a control group receiving conventional therapy.[169] However, IVIG may offer benefit in the management of HIV-associated ITP in adults. Here, a dose of 1–2 g/kg per day for 2–5 days is recommended.[146]

Neurological diseases Chronic inflammatory demyelinating polyneuropathy (CIDP) is considered to be the chronic variety of the Guillain–Barré syndrome. CIDP is a treatable disorder. In several trials, IVIGs have proved to be effective in improving the clinical symptoms of this disease.[170–172] The proportion of CIDP patients who respond to IVIG treatment seems to depend on selection criteria. Especially patients who have signs of active disease with involvement of both arms and legs have a chance to improve after IVIG therapy.[173] About 75% of patients who initially respond need intermittent IVIG infusions for several years. However, the best treatment for CIDP is still not known. Besides IVIGs, steroids and plasma exchange are effective in the majority of patients.[174] A trial comparing plasma exchange and IVIGs suggested that they have a similar effect.[175] A clinical trial directly comparing IVIGs with steroids has not been published. Moreover, CIDP is a chronic disease; no trial has been published evaluating the effects of long-term IVIG treatment.

Experimental indications

In these diseases there may be case reports showing the benefits of IVIG treatment in selected patients, or theoretical considerations suggesting some potential beneficial effects of IVIG, but well-performed, controlled clinical studies are lacking. IVIG treatment may be considered as a last resort, and patients should be informed about the experimental nature of treatment. Research is required to provide a more rational basis for IVIG treatment, e.g. by finding diagnostic criteria to identify subsets of patients who may be responsive to IVIG, and criteria to assess the therapeutic effects.

Neurological diseases

IVIGs have been investigated as a last-resort therapy in various neurological diseases in patients unresponsive to other therapies. Most of the studies have been small-scale, however, and criteria for identification of subsets of patients who may be responsive to IVIG have not been established. Further research will be necessary to clarify the role of IVIGs in neurological diseases such as multiple sclerosis, intractable seizure disorders,[176,177] myasthenia gravis,[178,179] and others.

In myasthenia gravis, one randomized controlled trial compared IVIGs with plasma exchange in a group of 87 patients suffering an acute exacerbation.[180] A similar degree of improvement was observed for both treatments. However, placebo-controlled clinical trials are still lacking to prove clinical benefit. In multiple sclerosis, several uncontrolled or open-label studies suggest a beneficial effect of IVIGs on the course of the disease.[181,182] In a placebo-controlled trial, Fazekas et al[183] proved that IVIGs have a significant effect on the course of clinical disability in patients with relapsing–remitting multiple sclerosis.

Burn injuries

Following a severe burn, all components of the immune system are suppressed. Serum immunoglobulin levels are low, because of capillary leakage and increased catabolism, and the natural barrier against infection—the skin—is destroyed. This makes patients with severe thermal injury highly susceptible to infection. However, decreases in mortality and incidence of sepsis have not been demonstrated during IGIV treatment.[184]

Sepsis

Treatment of patients with Gram-negative bacteraemia and shock using a human antiserum to endotoxin of a mutant *E. coli* strain has been shown to be effective in a small study.[185] In a number of small studies IVIG administration has been shown to improve the outcome of patients with Gram-negative bacteraemia and septic shock.[186,187] However, beneficial effects could not be confirmed in larger-scale trials using either polyvalent IVIGs or an IgM-enriched preparation.[188–190] In one trial a strictly selected group of septic patients in whom circulating endotoxin levels could be detected profited from the administration of an IgM-enriched immunoglobulin preparation;[191] however, endotoxin detection is difficult and not routinely available. One problem of IVIGs in septic patients is that once septic shock is present IVIG treatment comes too late; on the other hand, prophylactic administration of IVIG to all patients at risk of developing septicaemia is expensive, and many patients will be treated unnecessarily. Differences in outcome between different clinical trials may be explained by differences in type and frequency of nosocomial infections between trial centres. Larger, controlled trials will be needed to establish which patients will profit from IVIG administration, as well as the cost-effectiveness of such measures.[192]

Autoimmune rheumatic disorders

IVIGs have been investigated in numerous small studies in diseases such as systemic lupus erythematosus, rheumatoid arthritis, juvenile chronic arthritis, polymyositis and dermatomyositis, ANCA-positive vasculitis and Sjögren syndrome. Although some patients seem to profit from such therapy, no general recommendation can be made for the use of IVIGs in these diseases. Dosages and treatment duration also need to be specified. However, IVIGs may be a choice as a last-resort therapy for severely affected patients in whom other treatment has failed.

Other diseases

Numerous other diseases with established or hypothesized immunological pathogenesis have been treated with IVIG. As the list of these diseases is growing longer, no attempt is made to discuss them all within this review. Success rates have generally been variable, and many reports were based on case reports or small uncontrolled studies. The decision to administer IVIG outside clinical trials should be carefully weighed against the potential risks, and be thoroughly discussed with the patient in each case.

Conclusion

Intravenous immunoglobulins are currently being used for a vast array of indications, many of which are not (or not yet) supported by data from controlled clinical trials. However, future studies will clarify the potential use of IVIG administration, and new indications will arise. As long as conclusive data are not available, IVIGs should be restrictively prescribed to patients in clinical routine, and clear outcome measures should be defined for each individual which will allow assessment of the patient's response to treatment. Once a preparation has been selected for a patient, the minimal risks of viral transmission and possible adverse reactions to immunoglobulin therapy should be discussed with the patient. Liver transaminase activities, serum creatinine concentration, and anti-IgA antibody titres (if indicated) should be measured at baseline.[66]

Commercially available IVIG products are prepared by variations of the original Cohn–Oncley process. While all modern products are subjected to virus inactivation procedures according to regulatory requirements, products may be different in other chemical, physical and pharmacological properties. Although all IVIG products may be considered therapeutically equivalent for primary immunodeficiency diseases and ITP, there may be important differences in therapeutic response in patients with other diseases. Comparing products for the purposes of formulary selection is therefore difficult. Therapeutic indications differ because clinical research performed with a particular IVIG product is often limited. Pharmaceutical properties and cost can be directly examined; however, direct comparisons between products have not been performed. Institutional decisions regarding formulary selection must therefore be made on the basis of required therapeutic indications, pharmaceutical and financial considerations, and patterns of institutional use and physician prescribing.

References

1. Cohn EJ, Strong LE, Hughes WL et al. Preparation and properties of serum and plasma protein. IV. A system for the separation into fractions of the protein and lipoprotein components of biological tissues and fluids. *J Am Chem Soc* 1946; **68**: 459–475.

2. Bruton OC. Agammaglobulinemia. *Pediatrics* 1952; **9**: 722–727.

3. Barandun S, Kisthler P, Jeunet F, Isliker H. Intravenous administration of human gammaglobulin. *Vox Sang* 1962; **7**: 157–174.

4. Janeway CA. The development of clinical uses of immunoglobulins: a review. In: Merler E, ed. *Immunoglobulins*. Washington: National Academy of Sciences, 1970, 3–14.

5. Nolte MT, Pirofsky B, Gerritz GA, Golding B. Intravenous immunoglobulin therapy for antibody deficiency. *Clin Exp Immunol* 1979; **36**: 237–243.

6. Pirofsky B. Intravenous immune globulin therapy in hypogammaglobulinemia: a review. *Am J Med* 1984; **76 (suppl 3A)**: 53–60.

7. Berkman SA, Lee ML, Gale RP. Clinical uses of intravenous immunoglobulins. *Ann Intern Med* 1990; **112**: 278–293.

8. Lever AM, Webster AD, Brown D, Thomas HC. Non-A, non-B hepatitis occurring in agammaglobulinaemic patients after intravenous immunoglobulin. *Lancet* 1984; **ii**: 1062–1064.

9. Schiff RI. Transmission of viral infections through intravenous immune globulin. *New Engl J Med* 1984; **331**: 1649–1650.

10. Böger RH, Bode-Böger SM, Frölich JC. Intravenöse Immunglobuline. Grundlagen, Auswahlkriterien und Indikationen für ihren prophylaktischen und therapeutischen Einsatz. *Med Klinik* 1995; **90**: 520–526.

11. Morell A, Terry WD, Waldman TA. Metabolic properties of IgG subclasses in man. *J Clin Invest* 1970; **49**: 673–680.

12. Skvaril F. Clinical relevance of IgG subclasses. In: Morell A, Nydegger UE, eds. *Clinical Use of Intravenous Immunoglobulins*. London: Academic Press, 1986, 37–44.

13. Natvig JB, Kunkel HG. Immunoglobulins: classes, subclasses, genetic variants, and idiotypes. *Adv Immunol* 1973; **16**: 1–22.

14. WHO. Appropriate uses of human immunoglobulin in clinical practice: Memorandum from an IUIS/WHO meeting. *Bull WHO* 1982; **60**: 43–47.

15. European Pharmacopoea. Immunglobulinum humanum normale ad usum intravenosum. *Pharm Europ* 1994; **2**: 5–16.

16. Bundesgesundheitsamt, Paul-Ehrlich-Institut—Bundesamt für Sera und Impfstoffe. Bekanntmachung über die Zulassung von Arzneimitteln. *Bundesanzeiger* 1994; **84**: 4.5.

17. Römer J, Morgenthaler JJ, Scherz R, Skvaril F. Characterization of various immunoglobulin preparations for intravenous application. I. Protein composition and antibody content. *Vox Sang* 1982; **42**: 62–73.

18. Skvaril F, Gardi A. Differences among available immunoglobulin preparations for

intravenous use. *Ped Infect Dis J* 1988; 7: 43–48.

19. Kistler P, Nitschmann H. Large scale production of human plasma fractions. *Vox Sang* 1962; 7: 414–419.

20. Debré M, Bonnet MC, Fridman WH et al. Infusion of Fcγ fragments for treatment of children with acute immune thrombocytopenic purpura. *Lancet* 1993; 342: 945–949.

21. Buckley RH, Schiff RI. The use of intravenous immune globulin in immunodeficiency diseases. *New Engl J Med* 1991; 325: 110–117.

22. Theobald K, Högy B. Pharmacokinetics of single and multiple infusions of 5S intravenous immunoglobulin. *Vox Sang* 1995; 68: 5–8.

23. Tankersley DL. Dimer formation in immunoglobulin preparations and speculations on the mechanism of action of intravenous immune globulin in autoimmune diseases. *Immunol Rev* 1994; 139: 159–172.

24. Morell A, Schurch B, Ryser D et al. In vivo behaviour of gamma globulin preparations. *Vox Sang* 1980; 38: 272–283.

25. Weisman LE, Stoll BJ, Kueser TJ et al. Intravenous immune globulin therapy for early-onset sepsis in premature neonates. *J Pediatr* 1992; 121: 434–443.

26. Noya FJ, Rench MA, Courbney JT et al. Pharmacokinetics of intravenous immunoglobulins in very low birth weight neonates. *Pediatr Infect Dis* 1989; 8: 759–763.

27. Kinney J, Mundorf L, Gleason C et al. Efficacy and pharmacokinetics of intravenous immune globulin administration to high-risk neonates. *Am J Dis Child* 1991; 145: 1233–1238.

28. Rand KH, Houck K, Ganju A et al. Pharmacokinetics of cytomegalovirus specific IgG antibody following intravenous immunoglobulin in bone marrow transplant patients. *Bone Marrow Transplant* 1989; 4: 679–683.

29. Lever AM, Yap PL, Cuthbertson B et al. Increased half-life of gammaglobulin after prolonged intravenous replacement therapy. *Clin Exp Immunol* 1987; 67: 441–446.

30. Thomas MJ, Brennan VM, Chapel HH. Rapid subcutaneous immunoglobulin infusion in children [letter]. *Lancet* 1993; 342: 1432–1433.

31. European Community. EC Directive on Self-Sufficiency in Blood Products (89/381/EEC), 1989.

32. Dawson GJ, Lesniewski RR, Stewart JL et al. Detection of antibodies to hepatitis C virus in US blood donors. *J Clin Microbiol* 1991; 29: 551–556.

33. Fiedler H. Seropositivity in paid blood donors. *Lancet* 1992; i: 551.

34. Kühnl P, Seidl S, Stangel W et al. Antibody to hepatitis C virus in German blood donors. *Lancet* 1989; ii: 324.

35. van der Poel CL, Reesink HW, Lelie PN et al. Anti-hepatitis C antibodies and non-A, non-B post transfusion hepatitis in the Netherlands. *Lancet* 1989; ii: 297–298.

36. Lindholm A. Epidemiology of viral infections in the Swedish blood-donor population. *Blood Coag Fibrinol* 1994; 5 (suppl 3): S13–S18.

37. Weber B, Rabenau H, Berger A et al. Seroprevalence of HCV, HAV, HBV, HDV, HCMV and HIV in high risk groups/Frankfurt a.M., Germany. *Zbl Bakt* 1995; 282: 102–112.

38. Dodd RY. Infectious risk of plasma donations:

relationship to safety of intravenous immune globulins. *Clin Exp Immunol* 1996; **104** (**suppl 1**): 31–34.

39. Mitra G, Wong MF, Mozen MM et al. Elimination of infectious retroviruses during preparation of immunoglobulins. *Transfusion* 1986; **26**: 394–397.

40. Wells MA, Wittek AE, Epstein JS et al. Inactivation and partition of human T-cell lymphotropic virus, type III, during ethanol fractionation of plasma. *Transfusion* 1986; **26**: 210–213.

41. Yei S, Yu MW, Tankersley DL. Partitioning of hepatitis C virus during Cohn-Oncley fractionation of plasma. *Transfusion* 1992; **32**: 824–828.

42. Yu MYW, Mason BL, Tankersley DL. Detection and characterization of hepatitis C virus RNA in immune globulin. *Transfusion* 1994; **34**: 596–602.

43. Lane RS. Non-A, non-B hepatitis from intravenous immunoglobulin. *Lancet* 1983; **ii**: 974–975.

44. Ochs HD, Fisher SH, Virant FS et al. Non-A, non-B hepatitis and intravenous immunoglobulin [letter]. *Lancet* 1985; **i**: 404–405.

45. Ochs HD, Fisher SH, Virant FS et al. Non-A, non-B hepatitis and intravenous immunoglobulin [letter]. *Lancet* 1986; **i**: 322–323.

46. Weiland O, Mattson L, Glaumann H. Non-A, non-B hepatitis and intravenous immunoglobulin. *Lancet* 1986; **i**: 976–977.

47. Hammarström L, Smith CIE. IgM production in hypogammaglobulinemic patients during non-A, non-B hepatitis. *Lancet* 1986; **i**: 743.

48. Björkander J, Cunningham-Rundles C, Lundin P et al. Intravenous immunoglobulin prophylaxis causing liver damage in 16 of 77 patients with hypogammaglobulinemia or IgG subclass deficiency. *Am J Med* 1988; **84**: 107–111.

49. Williams PE, Yap PL, Gillon J et al. Transmission of non-A, non-B hepatitis by pH4-treated intravenous immunoglobulin. *Vox Sang* 1989; **57**: 15–18.

50. Bjoro K, Froland SS, Yun Z et al. Hepatitis C infection in patients with primary hypogammaglobulinemia after treatment with contaminated immune globulin. *New Engl J Med* 1994; **331**: 1607–1611.

51. Yap PL, McOmish F, Webster ADB et al. Hepatitis C virus transmission by intravenous immunoglobulin. *J Hepatol* 1994; **21**: 455–460.

52. Bresee JS, Mast EE, Coleman PJ et al. Hepatitis C virus infection associated with administration of intravenous immune globulin. *J Am Med Assoc* 1996; **276**: 1563–1567.

53. Yap PL. The viral safety of intravenous immune globulin. *Clin Exp Immunol* 1996; **104** (**suppl I**): 35–42.

54. Commission of the European Community. Validation of virus removal and inactivation procedures. 1991. III/8115/89-EN-Final 1991.

55. Hamamoto Y, Harada S, Yamamoto N et al. Elimination of viruses (human immunodeficiency, hepatitis B, vesicular stomatitis and sindbis viruses) from an intravenous immunoglobulin preparation. *Vox Sang* 1987; **53**: 65–69.

56. Uemura Y, Uriyu K, Hirao Y et al. Inactivation and elimination of viruses during the fractionation of an intravenous immunoglobulin preparation: liquid heat treatment and polyethylene glycol fractionation. *Vox Sang* 1989; **56**: 155–161.

57. Reid KG, Cuthbertson B, Jones ADL, McIntosh RV. Potential contribution of mild pepsin treatment at pH4 to the viral safety of human immunoglobulin products. *Vox Sang* 1988; **55**: 75–80.

58. Kempf C, Jentsch P, Poirier B et al. Virus inactivation during production of intravenous immunoglobulin. *Transfusion* 1991; **31**: 423–427.

59. Eriksson B, Westman L, Jernberg M. Virus validation of plasma-derived products produced by Pharmacia, with particular reference to immunoglobulins. *Blood Coag Fibrinol* 1994; **5** (suppl 3): S37–S44.

60. Dichtelmüller H, Rudnick D, Breuer B, Gänshirt KH. Validation of virus inactivation and removal for the manufacturing procedure of two immunoglobulins and a 5% serum protein solution treated with β-propiolactone. *Biologicals* 1993; **21**: 259–268.

61. Horowitz B, Prince AM, Hamman J, Watklevicz C. Viral safety of solvent/detergent-treated blood products. *Blood Coag Fibrinol* 1994; **5** (suppl 3): S21–S28.

62. Yang YHJ, Ngo C, Yeh IN, Uemura Y. Antibody Fc functional activity of intravenous immunoglobulin preparations treated with solvent-detergent for virus inactivation. *Vox Sang* 1994; **67**: 337–344.

63. Stephan W, Dichtelmüller H, Prince AM et al. Inactivation of the Hutchinson strain of hepatitis non-A, non-B virus in intravenous immunoglobulin by beta-propiolactone. *J Med Virol* 1988; **26**: 227–232.

64. Zuhrie SR, Webster ADB, Davies R et al. A prospective controlled crossover trial of a new heat-treated intravenous immunoglobulin. *Clin Exp Immunol* 1995; **99**: 10–15.

65. Hanley JA, Lippman-Hand A. If nothing goes wrong, is everything all right? *JAMA* 1983; **249**: 1743–1745.

66. Chapel HM, Consensus Panel for the Diagnosis and Management of Primary Antibody Deficiencies. Consensus on diagnosis and management of primary antibody deficiencies. *Br Med J* 1994; **308**: 581–585.

67. Schiff RI. Intravenous gammaglobulin: pharmacology, clinical uses and mechanisms of action. *Pediatr Allergy Immunol* 1994; **5**: 63–87.

68. Day NK, Good RA, Wahn V. Adverse reactions in selected patients following intravenous infusions of gamma globulin. *Am J Med* 1984; **76**: 25–32.

69. Burks AW, Sampson HA, Buckley RH. Anaphylactic reactions after gammaglobulin administration in patients with hypogammaglobulinemia. Detection of IgE antibodies to IgA. *New Engl J Med* 1986; **314**: 560–564.

70. Björkander J, Hammarstrom J, Smith CIE et al. Immunoglobulin prophylaxis in patients with antibody deficiency syndromes and anti-IgA antibodies. *J Clin Immunol* 1987; **7**: 8–15.

71. Bleeker WK, Agterberg J, Ritger G et al. Key role of macrophages in hypotensive side effects of immunoglobulin preparations. Studies in an animal model. *Clin Exp Immunol* 1989; **77**: 338–344.

72. Misbah S, Chapel HM. Adverse effects of immunoglobulin therapy. *Drug Safety* 1993; **9**: 254–262.

73. Sacher RA. Intravenous gammaglobulin products: Development, pharmacology and precautions. In: Garner RJ, Sacher RA, eds. *Intravenous Gammaglobulin Therapy.* Arlington, VA: American Association of Blood Banks, 1988, 1–30.

74. Gelfand EW. Intravenous gammaglobulin therapy in immunocompromised patients. In: Garner RJ, Sacher RA, eds. *Intravenous Gammaglobulin Therapy.* Arlington, VA: American Association of Blood Banks, 1988, 31–46.

75. Roberton DM, Hosking CS. Use of methylprednisolone as prophylaxis for immediate adverse reactions in hypogammaglobulinaemic patients receiving intravenous immunoglobulin: A controlled trial. *Aust Paediatr J* 1988; **24**: 174–177.

76. Rodeghiero F, Castaman G, Vespignani M et al. Erythema multiforme after intravenous immunoglobulin. *Blut* 1988; **56**: 145.

77. Casteels-van Daele M, Wijndaele L, Hunnink K. Intravenous immune globulin and acute aseptic meningitis. *New Engl J Med* 1990; **323**: 614–615.

78. Sekul EA, Cupler EJ, Dalakas MC. Aseptic meningitis associated with high-dose intravenous immunoglobulin therapy: frequency and risk factors. *Ann Intern Med* 1994; **121**: 259–262.

79. Frame WD, Crawford RJ. Thrombotic events after intravenous immunoglobulin. *Lancet* 1986; **ii**: 468.

80. Wooddruff RJ, Grigg AP, Firkin FC, Smith IL. Fatal thrombotic events during treatment of autoimmune thrombocytopenia with intravenous immunoglobulin in elderly patients. *Lancet* 1986; **ii**: 217–218.

81. Silbert PL, Knezevic WV, Bridge DT. Cerebral infarction complicating intravenous immunoglobulin for polyneuritis cranialis. *Neurology* 1992; **42**: 257–258.

82. Nakamura S, Yoshida T, Ohtake S, Matsuda T. Hemolysis due to high-dose intravenous immunoglobulin treatment for patients with idiopathic thrombocytopenic purpura. *Acta Haematol* 1986; **76**: 115–118.

83. Pisani G, Wirz M, Gentili G. Anti-D testing in intravenous immunoglobulins: shouldn't it be considered? *Vox Sang* 1996; **71**: 132.

84. Siber GR, Werner BG, Halsley NA et al. Interference of immune globulin with measles and rubella immunization. *J Pediatr* 1993; **122**: 204–211.

85. Alving BM, Tankersley DL, Mason BL et al. Contact-activated factors: contaminants of immunoglobulin preparations with coagulant and vasoactive properties. *J Lab Clin Med* 1980; **96**: 334–346.

87. Ahsan N, Palmer BF, Wheeler D et al. Intravenous immunoglobulin-induced osmotic nephrosis. *Arch Intern Med* 1994; **154**: 1985–1987.

88. Schifferli J, Leski M, Favre H et al. High-dose intravenous IgG treatment and renal function. *Lancet* 1991; **337**: 457–458.

89. Bertorini TE, Nance AM, Horner LH et al. Complications of intravenous gammaglobulin in neuromuscular and other diseases. *Muscle Nerve* 1996; **19**: 388–391.

90. Sultan Y, Kazatchkine MD, Maissonnguue P, Nydegger UE. Anti-idiotypic suppression of autoantibodies in factor VIII (anti-hemophilic factor) by high dose intravenous immunoglobulin. *Lancet* 1984; **ii**: 765–768.

91. Rossi F, Sultan J, Kazatchkine MD. Spontaneous and therapeutic suppression of autoimmune response to factor VIII by anti-idiotypic antibodies. In: Morell A, Nydegger UE, eds. *Clinical Use of Intravenous Immunoglobulins.* London: Academic Press, 1986, 420–430.

92. Bussel J. Hilgartner MW. The use and mechanism of action of intravenous immunoglobulin in the treatment of immune haematologic disease. *Br J Haematol* 1984; **56**: 1–7.

93. Kelton JG. The interaction of IgG with reticuloendothelial cells: biological and therapeutic implications. In: Garatty G, ed. *Current Concepts in Transfusion Therapy.* Arlington, VA: American Association of Blood Banks, 1985, 51–107.

94. Mannhalter JW, Eibl MM. Down regulation of Fc receptors by IVIgG. *Int Rev Immunol* 1989; **5**: 173–179.

95. Delfraissy JF, Tchernia G, Laurian Y et al. Suppressor cell function after intravenous gamma globulin treatment in adult chronic idiopathic thrombocytopenic purpura. *Br J Haematol* 1985; **60**: 315–322.

96. Basta M, Fries LF, Frank MM. High doses of intravenous Ig inhibit in vitro uptake of C4 fragments onto sensitized erythrocytes. *Blood* 1991; **77**: 376–380.

97. Basta M, Kirshbom P, Frank MM, Fries LF. Mechanism of therapeutic effect of high-dose intravenous immunoglobulin. Attenuation of acute complement-dependent immune damage in a guinea pig model. *J Clin Invest* 1989; **84**: 1974–1981.

98. Schifferli JA, Didierjean L, Saurat JH. Immunomodulatory effects of intravenous immunoglobulin G. *J Rheumatol* 1991; **18**: 937–939.

99. Andersson J, Skansen-Saphir U, Sparrelid E, Andersson U. Intravenous immune globulin affects cytokine production in T lymphocytes and monocytes/macrophages. *Clin Exp Immunol* 1996; **104 (suppl 1)**: 10–20.

100. Kondo N, Ozawa T, Mushiake K et al. Suppression of immunoglobulin production of lymphocytes by intravenous immunoglobulin. *J Clin Immunol* 1990; **11**: 152–158.

101. Toyoda M, Zhang X, Petrosian A et al. Modulation of immunoglobulin production and cytokine mRNA expression in peripheral blood mononuclear cells by intravenous immunoglobulin. *J Clin Immunol* 1994; **14**: 178–189.

102. Mouthon L, Kaveri S, Kazatchkine M. Immune modulating effects of intravenous immunoglobulin (IVIg) in autoimmmune diseases. *Transfus Sci* 1994; **15**: 393–408.

103. Rubin RH, Fishman AK, Callahan RJ et al. ^{111}In-labeled nonspecific immunoglobulin scanning in the detection of focal infection. *New Engl J Med* 1989; **321**: 935–940.

104. Roux KH, Tankersley DL. A view of the human idiotypic repertoire. Electron microscopic and immunologic analyses of spontaneous idiotype-anti-idiotype dimers in pooled human IgG. *J Immunol* 1990; **144**: 1387–1395.

105. Mouthon L, Kaveri SV, Spalter SH et al. Mechanisms of action of intravenous immune globulin in immune-mediated diseases. *Clin Exp Immunol* 1996; **104 (suppl 1)**: 3–9.

106. Chapel HM, Consensus Panel for the Diagnosis and Management of Primary Antibody Deficiencies. *Consensus document for the diagnosis and management of patients with primary antibody deficiencies.* London: Royal College of Pathologists, 1995.

107. Cunningham-Rundles C. Clinical and immunologic analysis of 103 patients with common variable immunodeficiency. *J Clin Immunol* 1989; **9**: 22–33.

108. Hanson LA, Söderström R, Friman V et al. Update on IgA and IgG subclass deficiency. In: Chapel HM, Levinsky RJ, Webster ADB, eds. *Progress in Immune Deficiency III.* London: Royal Society of Medicine, 1991, 1–6.

109. Hermaszewskki RA, Webster ABD. Primary hypogammaglobulinemia: a survey of clinical manifestations and complications. *Quart J Med* 1993; **86**: 31–42.

110. Björkander J, Blake B, Hanson LA. Primary hypogammaglobulinemia: impaired lung function and body growth with delayed diagnosis and inadequate treatment. *Eur J Respir Dis* 1984; **65**: 529–536.

111. Medical Research Council. Hypogammaglobulinaemia in the United Kingdom. *Lancet* 1969; **i**: 163–168.

112. Garbett ND, Currie DC, Cole PJ. Comparison of the clinical efficacy and safety of an intramuscular and an intravenous immunoglobulin preparation for replacement therapy in idiopathic adult onset panhypogammaglobulinemia. *Clin Exp Immunol* 1989; **76**: 1–7.

113. Roifman CM, Levison H, Gelfand EW. High-dose versus low-dose intravenous immunoglobulin in hypogammaglobulinemia and chronic lung disease. *Lancet* 1987; **i**: 1075–1077.

114. Amman AJ, Ashman RF, Buckley RH et al. Use of intravenous gamma-globulin in antibody immunodeficiency: results of a multicenter controlled trial. *Clin Immunol Immunpathol* 1982; **22**: 60–67.

115. Montanaro A, Pirofsky B. Prolonged interval high-dose intravenous immunoglobulin in patients with primary immunodeficiency states. *Am J Med* 1984; **76**: 67–72.

116. Gelfand EW, Reid B, Roifman CM. Intravenous immune serum globulin replacement in hypogammaglobulinemia. A comparison of high-versus low-dose therapy. *Monogr Allergy* 1988; **23**: 177–186.

117. Hanson LA, Söderström R, Avanzini A et al. Immunoglobulin subclass deficiency. *Pediatr Infect Dis* 1988; 7 (**suppl**): S17–S21.

118. Aucouturier P, Lacombe C, Bremard C et al. Serum IgG subclass levels in patients with primary immunodeficiency syndromes or abnormal susceptibility to infections. *Clin Immunol Immunpathol* 1989; **51**: 22–37.

119. Bass JL, Nuss R, Mehta KA, Morganelli P, Bennett L. Recurrent meningococcemia associated with IgG2 subclass deficiency [letter]. *New Engl J Med* 1983; **309**: 430.

120. Gross S, Blaiss MS, Herrod HG. Role of immunoglobulin subclasses and specific antibody determinations in the evaluation of recurrent infection in children. *J Pediatr* 1992; **121**: 516–522.

121. Umetsu DT, Ambrosino DM, Quinti I et al. Recurrent sinopulmonary infection and impaired antibody response to bacterial capsular polysaccharide antigen in children with selective IgG subclass deficiency. *New Engl J Med* 1985; **313**: 1247–1251.

122. Ambrosino DM, Umetsu DT, Siber GR et al. Selective defect in the antibody response to *Haemophilus influenzae* type b in children with recurrent infections and normal IgG subclass levels. *J Allergy Clin Immunol* 1988; **81**: 1175–1179.

123. Silk HJ, Ambrosino D, Geha RS. Effect of intravenous gammaglobulin therapy in IgG2 deficient and IgG2 sufficient children with recurrent infections and poor response to immunization with *Haemophilus influenzae* Type b capsular polysaccharide antigen. *Ann Allergy* 1990; **64**: 21–25.

124. Björkander J, Bengtsson U, Oxelius V, Hanson LA. Symptoms in patients with lowered levels of IgG subclasses, with or without IgA deficiency, and effects of immunoglobulin prophylaxis. *Monogr Allergy* 1986; **20**: 157–163.

125. Hanson LA, Söderström R, Nilssen DE et al. IgG subclass deficiency with or without IgA deficiency. *Clin Immunol Immunpathol* 1991; **61** (**suppl**): S70–S77.

126. Blaese SM, Strober W, Waldmann TA. Immunodeficiency in the Wiskott-Aldrich syndrome. *Birth Def* 1975; **11**: 250–254.

127. Boder E. Ataxia-telangiectasia: an overview. In: *Ataxia-telangiectasia: Genetics, Neuropathology, and Immunology of a Degenerative Disease of Childhood*. New York: Liss, 1985, 1–63.

128. Sullivan JL, Woda BA. X-linked lymphoproliferative syndrome. *Immunodef Rev* 1989; **1**: 325–347.

129. Ferrieri P. Neonatal susceptibility and immunity to major bacterial pathogens. *J Infect Dis* 1990; **12** (**suppl**): S394–S400.

130. Sidiropoulos D, Boehme U, Muralt G et al. Immunoglobulin supplementation in prevention or treatment of neonatal sepsis. *Pediatr Infect Dis* 1986; **5** (**suppl**): S193–S194.

131. Clapp DW, Kliegman RM, Baley JE et al. Use of intravenously administered immune globulin to prevent nosocomial sepsis in low birth weight infants: report of a pilot study. *J Pediatr* 1989; **115**: 973–978.

132. Bussel JB. Intravenous gammaglobulin in the prophylaxis of late sepsis in very-low-birth-weight infants: preliminary results of a randomized double-blind, placebo-controlled trial. *Rev Infect Dis* 1990; **12** (**suppl**): S457–S462.

133. Baker CJ, Melish ME, Hall RT et al. Intravenous immune globulin for the prevention of nosocomial infection in low-birth-weight neonates. *New Engl J Med* 1992; **327**: 213–219.

134. Zbrozek AS. The cost of cytomegalovirus disease in renal transplantation [letter]. *Transplantation* 1994; **57**: 165.

135. Chou S. Acquisition of donor-strains of cytomegalovirus by renal transplant recipients. *New Engl J Med* 1986; **314**: 1418–1423.

136. Wreghitt TG, Hakim M, Gray JJ et al. Cytomegalovirus infections in heart and heart and lung transplant recipients. *J Clin Pathol* 1988; **41**: 660–667.

137. Snydman DR. Cytomegalovirus immunoglobulins in the prevention and treatment of cytomegalovirus disease. *Rev Infect Dis* 1990; **12** (**suppl**): S839–S848.

138. Conti DJ, Freed BM, Lempert N. Prophylactic immunoglobulin therapy improves the outcome of renal transplantation in recipients at risk for primary cytomegalovirus disease. *Transplant Proc* 1993; **25**: 1421–1422.

139. Cremer J, Behrend M, Wahlers T et al. CMV-Infektionen nach Lungen- und Herz-Lungen-Transplantation. *Z Transplantationsmed* 1992; **4**: 60–64.

140. Müller R, Gubernatis M, Farle M et al. Liver transplantation in HBs antigen (HBsAg) carriers: prevention of hepatitis B virus (HBV) recurrence by passive immunization. *J Hepatol* 1991; **13**: 90–96.

141. Tutschka PJ. Infections and immunodeficiency in bone marrow transplantation. *Pediatr Infect Dis J* 1988; 7 (**suppl**): S22–S29.

142. Lenarsky C. Mechanisms in immune recovery after bone marrow transplantation. *Am J Pediatr Hem Onc* 1993; **15**: 49–55.

143. Winston DJ, Ho WG, Champlin RE, Gale RP. Infectious complications of bone marrow transplantation. *Int Soc Exp Hematol* 1984; **12**: 205–215.

144. Meyers JD, Flournoy N, Thomas ED. Risk factors for cytomegalovirus infection after human bone marrow transplantation. *J Infect Dis* 1986; **153**: 478–488.

145. NIH Consensus Conference. Intravenous immunoglobulin. Prevention and treatment of disease. *JAMA* 1990; **264**: 3189–3193.

146. ASHP Commission on Therapeutics. ASHP therapeutic guidelines for intravenous immune globulin. *Clin Pharm* 1992; **11**: 117–136.

147. Schmidt GM, Kovacs A, Zaia JA et al. Gancyclovir/immunoglobulin combination therapy for the treatment of human cytomegalovirus-associated interstitial pneumonia in bone marrow allograft recipients. *Transplantation* 1988; **46**: 905–907.

148. Sullivan KM. Immunoglobulin therapy in bone marrow transplantation. *Am J Med* 1987; **83**: 34–45.

149. Bass EB, Powe NR, Goodman SN et al. Efficacy of immune globulin in preventing complications of bone marrow transplantation: a meta-analysis. *Bone Marrow Transplant* 1993; **12**: 273–282.

150. Guglielmo BJ, Wong-Beringer A, Linker CA. Immune globulin therapy in allogeneic bone marrow transplant: a critical review. *Bone Marrow Transplant* 1994; **13**: 499–510.

151. Sullivan KM, Storek J, Kopecky KJ et al. A controlled trial of long-term administration of intravenous immunoglobulin to prevent late infection and chronic graft-vs.-host disease after marrow transplantation: clinical outcome and effect on subsequent immune recovery. *Biol Bone Marrow Transplant* 1996; **2**: 44–53.

152. National Institute of Child Health and Human Development Intravenous Immunoglobulin Study Group. Intravenous immune globulin for the prevention of bacterial infections in children with symptomatic human immunodeficiency virus infection. *New Engl J Med* 1991; **325**: 73–80.

153. Imbach P, Barandun S, d'Apuzzo V et al. High-dose intravenous gammaglobulin for idiopathic thrombocytopenic purpura in childhood. *Lancet* 1981; **i**: 1228–1230.

154. Karpatkin S. Autoimmune thrombocytopenic purpura. *Blood* 1980; **56**: 329–343.

155. Stiehm ER. Recent progress in the use of intravenous immunoglobulin. *Curr Probl Pediatr* 1992; **22**: 335–348.

156. Kawasaki T. Acute febrile mucocutaneous syndrome with lymphoid involvement with specific desquamation of the fingers and toes. *Jpn J Allergy* 1967; **16**: 178–222.

157. Melish ME. Kawasaki syndrome (the mucocutaneous lymph node syndrome). *Pediatr Ann* 1982; **11**: 255–268.

158. Newburger JW, Takahashi M, Burns JC et al. The treatment of Kawasaki syndrome with intravenous gamma globulin. *New Engl J Med* 1986; **315**: 341–347.

159. Newburger JW, Takahashi M, Beiser AS et al. A single intravenous infusion of gamma globulin as compared with four infusions in the treatment of acute Kawasaki syndrome. *New Engl J Med* 1991; **324**: 1633–1639.

160. Shahar E, Murphy EG, Roifman CM. Benefit of intravenously administered immune serum globulin in patients with Guillain–Barré syndrome. *J Pediatr* 1990; **116**: 141–144.

161. Van der Meché FGA, Schmitz PIM, Dutch Guillain–Barré Study Group. A randomized trial comparing intravenous immune globulin and plasma exchange in Guillain Barré syndrome. *New Engl J Med* 1992; **326**: 1123–1129.

162. Plasma Exchange/Sandoglobulin Guillain–Barré Trial Group. Randomised trial of plasma exchange, intravenous immunoglobulin, and combined treatments in

Guillain–Barré syndrome. *Lancet* 1997; **349**: 225–230.

163. Keller T, McGrath K, Newland A et al. Indications for use of intravenous immunoglobulin. *Med J Aust* 1993; **159**: 204–206.

164. Cooperative Group for the Study of Immunoglobulin in Chronic Lymphocytic Leukemia. Intravenous immunoglobulin for the prevention of infection in chronic lymphocytic leukemia: a randomized, controlled trial. *New Engl J Med* 1988; **319**: 902–907.

165. Schedel I. Application of immunoglobulin preparations in multiple myeloma. In: Morell A, Nydegger UE, eds. *Clinical Use of Intravenous Immunoglobulins*. New York: Academic Press, 1986, 123–132.

166. Schmidt RE, Hartlapp JH, Niese D et al. Reduction of infection frequency by intravenous gammaglobulin during intensive induction therapy for small-cell carcinoma of the lung. *Infection* 1984; **12**: 167–170.

167. Weeks JC, Tierney MR, Weinstein MC. Cost effectiveness of prophylactic intravenous immune globulin in chronic lymphocytic leukemia. *New Engl J Med* 1991; **325**: 81–86.

168. Ratko TA, Burnett DA, Foulke GE et al. Recommendations for off-label use of intravenously administered immunoglobulin preparations. *JAMA* 1995; **273**: 1865–1870.

169. Kiehl MG, Stoll R, Broder M et al. A controlled trial of intravenous immune globulin for the prevention of serious infections in adults with advanced human immunodeficiency virus infection. *Arch Intern Med* 1996; **156**: 2545–2550.

170. Van Doorn PA, Brand A, Strengers PFW et al. High-dose intravenous immunoglobulin treatment in chronic inflammatory demyelinating polyneuropathy. A double-blind, placebo-controlled crossover study. *Neurology* 1990; **40**: 209–212.

171. Vermeulen M, van Doorn PA, Brand A et al. Intravenous immunoglobulin treatment in patients with chronic inflammatory demyelinating polyneuropathy. A double-blind, placebo controlled study. *J Neurol Neurosurg Psych* 1993; **56**: 36–39.

172. Hahn AF, Bolton CF, Zochodne D, Feasby TE. Intravenous immunoglobulin treatment in chronic inflammatory demyelinating polyneuropathy. A double-blind, placebo-controlled crossover study. *Brain* 1996; **199**: 1067–1077.

173. van Doorn PA, Vermeulen M, Brand A et al. Intravenous immunoglobulin treatment in patients with chronic inflammatory demyelinating polyneuropathy. Clinical and laboratory characteristics associated with improvement. *Arch Neurol* 1991; **48**: 217–220.

174. Van der Meché FGA, van Doorn PA. Guillain–Barré syndrome and chronic inflammatory demyelinating polyneuropathy: immune mechanisms and update on current therapies. *Ann Neurol* 1995; **37 (suppl 1)**: S14–S31.

175. Dyck PJ, Litchy WJ, Kratz KM, et al. A plasma exchange versus immune globulin infusion trial in chronic inflammatory demyelinating polyradiculoneuropathy. *Ann Neurol* 1994; **36**: 838–845.

176. Duse M, Tiberti S, Plebani A et al. IgG2 deficiency and intractable epilepsy of childhood. *Monogr. Allergy* 1986; **20**: 128–134.

177. Plebani A, Duse M, Tiberti S et al. Intravenous γ globulin therapy and serum

IgG subclass levels in intractable childhood epilepsy. *Monogr Allergy* 1988; **23**: 204–215.

178. Fateh-Moghadan A, Wick M, Besinger U, Geursen RG. High-dose intravenous gammaglobulin for myasthenia gravis. *Lancet* 1984; **i**: 848–849.

179. Sakano T, Hamasaki T, Kinoshita Y et al. Treatment for refractory myasthenia gravis. *Arch Dis Child* 1989; **64**: 1191–1193.

180. Gajdos P, Chevrer S, Clair B et al. Clinical trial of plasma exchange and high-dose intravenous gammaglobulin in myasthenia gravis. *Ann Neurol* 1997; **41**: 789–796.

181. Rothfelder U, Neu I, Pelka R. Therapy of multiple sclerosis with immunoglobulin. *Münch Med Wschr* 1982; **124**: 74–78.

182. Achiron A, Pras E, Cilad R et al. Open controlled therapeutic trial of intravenous immune globulin in relapsing-remitting multiple sclerosis. *Arch Neurol* 1992; **49**: 1233–1236.

183. Fazekas F, Deisenhammer F, Strasser-Fuchs S et al. Randomised placebo-controlled trial of monthly intravenous immunoglobulin therapy in relapsing-remitting multiple sclerosis. *Lancet* 1997; **349**: 589–593.

184. Waymack JP, Jenkins ME, Alexander JW et al. A prospective trial of prophylactic intravenous immune globulin for the prevention of infections in severely burned patients. *Burns* 1989; **15**: 71–76.

185. Ziegler EJ, McCutchan JA, Fierer J et al. Treatment of gram-negative bacteremia and shock with human antiserum to a mutant *Escherichia coli*. *New Engl J Med* 1982; **307**: 1225–1230.

186. Domimioni L, Diongi R, Zanello M et al. Effects of high-dose IgG on survival of surgical patients with sepsis scores of 20 or greater. *Arch Surg* 1991; **126**: 236–240.

187. Ziegler EJ, Fisher CJ, Sprung CL et al. Treatment of gram-negative bacteremia and septic shock with HA-1A human monoclonal antibody against endotoxin. *New Engl J Med* 1991; **324**: 429–436.

188. Jesdinsky HJ, Tempel G, Castrup HJ, Seifert J. Cooperative group of additional immunoglobulin therapy in severe bacterial infections: Results of a multicenter randomized controlled trial in cases of diffuse fibrin-opurulent peritonitis. *Klin Wschr* 1987; **65**: 1132–1138.

189. Seifert J, Nitsche D. Immunglobulin M. Eigenschaften, Wirksamkeit und klinischer Nutzen. *Dtsch Med Wschr* 1987; **112**: 1267–1271.

190. De Simone C, Delogou G, Corbetta G. Intravenous immunoglobulins in association with antibiotics: a therapeutical trial in septic intensive care unit patients. *Crit Care Med* 1988; **16**: 23–26.

191. Schedel I, Dreikhausen U, Nentwig B et al. Treatment of gram-negative septic shock with an immunoglobulin preparation: a prospective, randomized clinical trial. *Crit Care Med* 1991; **19**: 1104–1113.

192. Werdan K, Pilz G. Supplemental immune globulins in sepsis: a critical appraisal. *Clin Exp Immunol* 1996; **104** (**suppl 1**): 83–90.

Safety and tolerability of intravenous immunoglobulins

Turf D Martin

12

> HAV: hepatitis A virus; HIV: human immunodeficiency virus; HTLV-I: human T-cell lymphotropic virus type I; Ig: immunoglobulin; IVIG: intravenous immunoglobulin; PCR: polymerase chain reaction

Introduction

Intravenous immunoglobulin (IVIG) is derived from human plasma by recovery from whole blood donors or by plasmapheresis. Prior to 1981, only products that had incomplete Fc function were commercially available from manufacturers. These products were used in a limited manner for immune replacement in patients with defective IgG. The second-generation products with an intact Fc function have allowed the use of IVIG for broader immune replacement therapy in patients with defective B-cell function and in immune modulation. This has resulted in the significant increase in the use of IVIG in autoimmune disorders, including those in neurology. Current applications include central nervous disorders such as remitting–relapsing multiple sclerosis, and peripheral nerve disorders such as chronic inflammatory demyelinating polyneuropathies, Guillain–Barré syndrome, multifocal motor neuropathies, polymyositis and myasthenia gravis.

Virological safety

Because IVIG is a plasma derivative, concern has been expressed about the potential for virus transmission. The viruses in question are the transfusion-related viruses such as hepatitis viruses A, B and C; human immunodeficiency virus; human T-cell lymphotropic virus types I and II; cytomegalovirus; human herpes virus; and parvovirus B-19. This became a major problem in 1994, following the reported transmission of hepatitis C in 247 patients receiving the IVIG product Gammagard (Baxter Healthcare Corporation, Hyland Division, Glendale, California, USA).[1] Reports of non-A, non-B hepatitis transmission have been published since 1983.[2–7] Other infections have recently caused concern, including Creutzfeldt–Jakob disease and hepatitis G.

Viral safety with IVIG begins with the donor and the donor center, i.e. the starting material. Within Europe and North America, all centers must meet either European Community (EC) or Food and Drug Administration (FDA) criteria. In North America, some donor centers qualify for a program administered by the American Blood Resources Organization called the Quality Plasma Program which sets higher standards than even those of the FDA. European manufacturers obtain their plasma from the USA and/or Europe (usually Austria and Germany, unless the company is nationally controlled). Many political agendas surround the issue of remunerated versus nonremunerated donors. The issue that appears important is that of the quality and certification of the donor centers. No difference in the safety, tolerability, or efficacy of products derived from one or the other type of donor center has been documented. Donor centers must maintain a high level of quality control in their testing laboratories, absolute matching of donor records with plasma donations (traceability) and provide virologic follow-up analysis. Donors are given a medical physical examination, a complicated life-style analysis to screen out potential high-risk donations, and virologic testing. Plasmapheresis donors are often repeat donors (>75%) and may donate more frequently than whole-blood donors. Some manufacturers prefer to use plasmapheresis donors in order to have greater standardization between lots of IVIG. All commercial products today are derived from more than 1000 donors per lot.

Appropriate screening of donors reduces the risks of viral transmission, but manufacturers must still employ methods of viral separation and inactivation to reduce the risk of viral transmission. The difficulty is that no single method of viral separation or inactivation is totally effective. Many manufacturers have only validated current purification methods, with respect to viral log reduction, without implementing more formal methods of destroying and/or eliminating viruses. Indeed, some manufacturers rely almost totally upon screening, e.g. polymerase chain reaction (PCR). Since 1 July 1999, hepatitis C antigen screening of the pooled plasma is a requirement of the European authorities. The Americans have required hepatitis C antigen screening by PCR since 1995 for products that lack a formal virus inactivation step. The basic problem with screening is that only known viruses may be screened for, and there is currently a lack of standardized testing methods and kits for most viruses. This lack of standardization results in different detection limits, false positives and false negatives. Besides the issue of detection limits, many assays are not validated by the assay manufacturers in the final products. The product itself or its excipients may cross-react, producing indeterminate or false results.

Three methods of primary viral inactivation are used by industry (*Table 12.1*). The use of solvent/detergent is extremely effective against lipid-coated viruses, e.g. hepatitis C,[8–10] but has little activity against nonlipid-coated viruses, e.g. parvovirus B-19. This method is gaining a wide acceptance within the industry and with governmental regulatory authorities. Pasteurization is employed by only a few manufacturers. It is effective against those viruses sensitive to heat treatment to 60 °C. However, this excludes many viruses. Further, the IgG molecule begins denaturation at 59–61 °C, thus requiring extremely tight manufacturing controls. Beta-propiolactone is employed by one manufacturer. This method appears to be the most effective against both lipid-coated and nonlipid-coated viruses, but unfortunately damages the Fc portion of the IgG molecule. Because no single primary method is totally effective, manufacturers employ additional secondary steps including incubation at pH 4, addition of pepsin, caprylic acid, polyethylene glycol, and hydrolase treatment. Viral separation techniques are also employed by some firms including nanofiltration, chromatography, and the Cohn-Oncley fractionation steps. Still some viruses are extremely difficult to remove or kill, e.g. parvovirus B-19. Therefore some firms set minimum standards of antibody levels against these antigens to ensure neutralization. The FDA and EC continue to examine this situation and propose new regulations. The

Table 12.1
Methods of viral inactivation and/or removal in the manufacture of intravenous immunoglobulin.

Primary inactivation methods	Secondary inactivation methods	Separation methods
Solvent/detergent Pasteurization β-Propiolactone	Incubation at pH 4 Caprylic acid Addition of pepsin Hydrolase treatment Polyethylene glycol Low pH storage	Cohn–Oncley fractionation Nanofiltration Column chromatography Ion exchange Neutralizing antibodies

German authorities proposed specific logarithmic reductions with multiple steps of inactivation in 1994.[11] These became only recommendations in 1995 after many members of industry and EC member states complained that compliance was not readily achievable. It is interesting to note that several companies are now able to comply with these stringent standards.

All three of the primary methods of inactivation are effective against hepatitis C virus and most lipid-coated viruses. The difficulty is with the inactivation and/or removal of nonlipid-coated viruses, e.g. hepatitis A virus (HAV) and parvovirus B-19. No effective process for the destruction of these viruses exists with today's commercial technology in IVIG. Both are susceptible to inactivation by exposure to high levels of heat treatment, e.g. 100 °C. Nanofiltration is only effective for the larger viruses as the smallest effective filter than can be used is 35 nm (the diameter of HAV is approximately 30 nm and that of parvovirus B-19 is 18–26 nm). Therefore it is critical to ensure that commercial IVIG preparations have adequate antibody levels of HAV and parvovirus B-19 to neutralize any antigen that may have contaminated the plasma pool. This neutralization process must be adequately validated by international standards.

Validation of these methods is only partially standardized. Laboratories use model viruses because they are unable to grow enough of the actual virus, e.g. hepatitis C. There is no uniformity of model viruses by all manufacturers and it is therefore very difficult to interpret between manufacturers' data. Clinicians should require manufacturers to provide clear and understandable data with respect to viral safety and should consult a virologist for interpretation of ambiguous information.

Tolerability

The increased utilization of IVIG in the therapy of autoimmune disorders has accentuated the issue of tolerability. The reported rate of adverse reactions with IVIG in clinical therapy ranges from 1% to 81%.[12,13] While the majority of adverse reactions are mild and related to the speed of infusion, an increasing number of more serious reactions are emerging with the use of higher doses: cerebral infarction, acute renal failure, aseptic meningitis, myocardial infarction, thrombosis, arthritis, hyperviscosity, and vasculitis. The difficulty in determining actual incidence is that most clinical studies are not designed to investigate tolerability, but rather to note adverse reactions. This has resulted in manufacturers reporting an incidence of 1% to 16% for adverse reactions in their official prescribing information. This information on tolerability is rarely updated after the initial registration unless mandated by a government authority. Only recently have authorities begun to require pharmacovigilance studies. Clinicians should inquire as to the availability of such a report from the manufacturer. Prior to this point, the only document(s) available were those which the companies were required to file, e.g. periodic safety reports and immediately notify government officials of any serious reactions. Octapharma AG, Lachen, Switzerland, has an ongoing post-market clinical pharmacovigilance study with its brand of IVIG, Octagam®. Results are available from 121 centers with 2554 treated patients and over 26 000 infusions during the last 4 years. The 4-year data demonstrate an adverse reaction rate of less than 0.5% for all patient infusions and less than 4% in all patients.

There does appear to be a significant difference between brands with respect to the global incidence of adverse reactions (*Table 12.2*). This may be due to a large variance in different pharmacological parameters between products. The majority of adverse reactions include headache, backache, nausea, vomiting, diarrhea, flushing, fever, chills, shaking, shortness of breath, tightness of the chest, hypotension, hypertension, and rashes. These are usually transitory in nature and related to the speed of the infusion. Different products have different rates of infusion because of differences in stabilizers, total protein content, pH and particle count. It is important that persons actually administering the IVIG read the manufacturer's package leaflet for the rate of infusion recommended for that specific product. These reactions usually occur within the first hour of the infusion. Should any of these reactions occur, stop the infusion, wait 30 minutes, and restart at a slower infusion speed. Even with the recommended infusion rate, a large interpatient variability exists such that some patients tolerate a much faster infusion speed while other patients require an

Table 12.2
Adverse reactions with intravenous immunoglobulins.

Mild	Moderate	Severe
Headache	Headache	Aseptic meningitis
Backache	Rashes	Acute renal failure
Nausea	Neutropenia	Cerebral infarction
Vomiting	Arthritis	Myocardial infarction
Diarrhea	Phlebitis	Hyperviscosity
Chills	Serum sickness	Thrombosis
Fever	Alopecia	Vasculitis
Shaking	Eczema	Hemolytic anemia
Flushing	Erythema multiforme	Disseminated intravascular
Hypertension	Leukopenia	coagulation
Hypotension	Anaphylactoid reactions	Anaphylaxis reaction
Tightness in the chest	Infusion site necrosis	
Shortness of breath		

even slower infusion speed. Some patients may react even with very slow infusion speeds and to different brands. These rare patients may require prophylactic treatment 30 minutes before IVIG infusion with 50–100 mg hydrocortisone, an antipyretic, and/or an antihistamine.[14,15]

With the exception of headache, which may occur up to 7 days after infusion, if these reactions occur at the end of the infusion or later they may be related to pyrogen contamination of the product. In vivo rabbit testing, required by regulatory authorities for product release for pyrogens, is limited in dosing to the equivalent of 200–600 mg/kg. Dosing for autoimmune disorders is frequently higher or more prolonged than for immune replacement. Therefore some manufacturers have instituted an in vitro *Limulus* test to look more closely for pyrogen contamination. Only testing in vivo is required by regulatory officials. These immediate reactions may also be due to rapid formation of immune complexes in patients who have never received IVIG or if more than 8 weeks have passed since the previous infusion. Additional reasons include the presence of aggregates, presence of fragments, insoluble or incompletely dissolved lyophilate (in products requiring mixing before administration), the temperature of the solution being infused, and the total protein load being administered (some products contain albumin in addition to the IgG).

Immunologic reasons may include triggering of an inflammatory response by product constituents, acute complement activation with production of anaphylatoxins C3a and C5a, triggering of mast cells and polymorphonuclear granulocytes resulting in the release of histamine and other granular components, and release of tumor necrosis factor and other interleukins.[12,16–20]

Another type of early adverse reaction is specific to products with a pH below 5.0. These products may produce severe irritation and/or necrosis at the infusion site. The package leaflets of two different brands report phlebitis and thrombotic complications. Neonates or those with impaired physiology may not be able to buffer the low pH adequately if large doses are required.

Severe headache has been documented in a number of neurologic patients.[21,22] Some headaches have been severe enough to require computed tomography scans, which showed no evidence of intracranial hemorrhage.[23] Patients prone to headache or delayed onset headache may require further slowing of the infusion speed or administration of low-dose beta-blockers, which has sometimes been effective.[14] Aseptic meningitis has been reported in up to 11% of neurologic patients receiving IVIG.[21] There is no evidence of subarachnoid hemorrhage, it is self-limiting, and without major sequelae. Elevated IgG levels of 1.5 to 7 times the upper limit of normal may be found in cerebrospinal fluid.[23]

Aseptic meningitis may mimic bacterial meningitis with neutrophilic pleocytosis, elevated protein concentration, and decreased glucose in the cerebrospinal fluid. Normal treatment is symptomatic with narcotic analgesics and antiemetics. However, some centers immediately begin antibiotic treatment because of the difficulty of differential diagnosis, and base treatment time on IgG clearance from the cerebrospinal fluid. Patients with a history of migraine appear to be at higher risk. The mechanism is unknown but may be due to a vasomotor effect on the meningeal microvasculature from an induced release of histamine, serotonin, or prostaglandins. Additional ideas are related to soluble molecules such as cytokines and human leukocyte antigens. The allogeneic IgG does cross the blood–brain barrier.

Arthritic complications have been described,[24] characterized by severe pain in several joints, especially the knees and wrists. Laboratory studies indicate elevated levels of circulating immune complexes as measured by binding to C3d, mild decrease in serum C4 levels and a mild increase in total hemolytic complement. Potential mechanisms of action include the formation of specific antibody–antigen immune complex aggregates and antiidiotypes directed against autoantibodies.

Acute renal failure is being seen more often with the high doses used in neurologic patients. The products implicated contain sucrose as a stabilizer and result in classical osmotic nephrosis.[22,25–27] Renal biopsy shows swelling and vacuolization of the proximal tubular epithelia cytoplasma, and IgG in the glomerulus. Creatinine levels may rise from 124 μmol/l (1.4 mg/dl) to more than 575 μmol/l (6.5 mg/dl). Besides the sucrose, the osmolality may be a potential complicating factor. Many manufacturers who produce lyophilized powders indicate that their products may be reconstituted at much higher concentrations than the standard 3% or 5%. At the standard concentrations, the osmolality is usually below 350 mosmol/kg. However, if a 6%, 10%, or 12% concentration is made from these products, osmolality may rise to over 1000 mosmol/kg. This, in combination with higher sodium content in some products, may present problems in patients with underlying renal complications, neonates, and patients over 60 years of age.

The osmolality issue may also be responsible for thrombogenesis secondary to hyperviscosity. Both cerebral infarction and myocardial infarction have been reported in older patients.[28–32] Plasma viscosity may rise by as much as 40%. Therefore it is not recommended to use products with an osmolality greater than 350 mosmol/kg in patients who may be sensitive to complications of hyperviscosity.

Additional complications have been associated with levels of isoagglutinins anti-A, anti-B, and anti-D. Products vary widely with regard to the content. Serum sickness without joint involvement and with immune hemolysis and disseminated intravascular coagulation has been reported, as well as hemolytic anemia.[33–35] Clinicians should request the content of isoagglutinins for the products prescribed.

Rare dermatologic events have been reported.[22] These include eczema, erythema multiforme, purpuric erythema, and alopecia. The mechanism for these is unknown but may be due to the presence of alloantibodies or antiidiotypes that form complexes with the patient's own alloantibodies.

Transient leukopenia[24] and neutropenia[36] have been reported. The leukopenia is normally asymptomatic. The neutropenia is rare. Proposed mechanisms of action include aggregates resulting in altered expression of cell surface CR3, thus causing adherence to blood vessels, the role of neutrophil FcRIII, and the presence in IVIG of antineutrophil antibodies.

Anaphylactic and anaphylactoid reactions with IVIG are rare. The majority of cases have been reported in immune-deficient patients treated with IVIG. The reaction is due to the formation of antibodies against IgA in patients who have no IgA. The mere presence of antibodies to IgA is not by itself indicative of the potential for anaphylaxis, but rather the rise in the IgA-Ab level prior to infusion. Product levels vary from 3 μg/ml to 8000 μg/ml.

Conclusion

The majority of adverse reactions are mild and easily managed, but clinicians need to be aware of the potential complications of IVIG, in regard to both viral safety and tolerability. Products vary significantly in their viral inactivation steps and pharmacological parameters. Clinicians should examine the choice of products carefully with respect to these issues before assuming that all IVIGs are generically the same. It appears that most IVIGs are equally efficacious, but the safety and tolerability vary widely which may result in severe morbidity and potential mortality.

References

1. Gomperts ED. Gammagard® and reported hepatitis C virus episodes. *Clin Ther* 1996; **18** (**suppl B**): 3–8.
2. Lane RS. Non-A non-B hepatitis from intravenous immunoglobulin. *Lancet* 1984; **2**: 974–975.
3. Lever AML, Webster ADB, Brown D, Thomas HC. Non-A, non-B hepatitis occurring in agammaglobulinaemic patients after intravenous immunoglobulin. *Lancet* 1984; 1062–1064.
4. Ochs HD, Fischer SH, Virant FS et al. Non-A, non-B hepatitis after intravenous immunoglobulin. *Lancet* 1985; **1**: 404–405.
5. Ochs, HD, Fischer SH, Virant FS et al. Non-A, non-B hepatitis after intravenous immunoglobulin [letter]. *Lancet* 1986; **1**: 323.
6. Björkander J, Cunningham-Rundles C, Lundin P et al. Intravenous immunoglobulin prophylaxis causing liver damage in 16 of 77 patients with hypogammaglobulinemia or IgG subclass deficiency. *Am J Med* 1988; **84**: 107–111.
7. Williams PE, Yap PL, Gillon J et al. Transmission of non-A, non-B hepatitis by pH 4.0 treated intravenous immunoglobulin. *Vox Sang* 1989; **57**: 15–18.
8. Horowitz B, Prince AM, Hamman J, Watklevicz C. Viral safety of solvent/detergent-treated products. *Blood Coag Fibrinol* 1994; **5** (**suppl 3**): S21–S28.
9. Eriksson B, Westman L, Jernberg M. Virus validation of plasma-derived products produced by Pharmacia, with particular reference to immunoglobulins. *Blood Coag Fibrinol* 1994; **5** (**suppl 3**): S37–S44.
10. Biesert L. Virus validation studies of immunoglobulin preparations. *Clin Exp Rheumatol* 1996; **14** (**suppl 15**): S47–S52.
11. Paul-Ehrlich Institut, Bundesamt für Sera und Impfstoffe. Notice relating to measures against drug-associated risks. Reduction of the risk of transmission of hematogenous viruses in case of drugs manufactured by fractionation of plasma of human origin. *Bundesanzeiger* 1994.
12. Weisman LE. The safety of intravenous immunoglobulin preparations. *Isr J Med Sci* 1994; **30**: 459–463.
13. Bertorini TE, Nance AM, Horner LH et al. Complications of intravenous gammaglobulin in neuromuscular and other diseases. *Muscle Nerve* 1996; **19**: 388–391.
14. Gelfand EW. Intravenous gammaglobulin therapy in immunocompromised patients. In: Garner RJ, Sacher RA, eds. *Intravenous Gammaglobulin Therapy*. Arlington, VA:

American Association of Blood Banks, 1988, 31–46.

15. Roberton DM, Hosking CS. Use of methylprednisolone as prophylaxis for immediate adverse infusion reactions in hypogammaglobulinaemic patients receiving intravenous immunoglobulin: a controlled trial. *Aust Paediatr J* 1988; **24**: 174–177.

16. Blaszcyk R, Westhoff V, Grosse-Wilde H. Soluble CD4, CD8 and HLA molecules in commercial immunoglobulin preparations. *Lancet* 1993; **341**: 789–790.

17. Lam L, Whitsett CF, McNichol JM, Hodge TW. Immunologically active proteins in intravenous immunoglobulin. *Lancet* 1992; **342**: 678.

18. Mollnes TE, Høgåsen K, Hoaas BF et al. Inhibition of complement-mediated red cell lysis by immmunoglobulins is dependent on the IG isotype and its C! binding properties. *Scand J Immunol* 1995; **41**: 449–456.

19. Mouthen L, Kaveri SV, Spalter SH et al. Mechanisms of action of intravenous immune globulin in immune-mediated diseases. *Clin Exp Immunol* 1996; **104 (suppl 1)**: 3–9.

20. Aukrust P, Müller F, Nordøy I et al. Modulation of lymphocyte and monocyte activity after intravenous immunoglobulin administration in vivo. *Clin Exp Immunol* 1997; **107**: 50–56.

21. Sekul EA, Cupler EJ, Dalakas MC. Aseptic meningitis associated with high-dose intravenous immunoglobulin therapy: frequency and risk factors. *Ann Intern Med* 1994; **121**: 259–262.

22. Brannagan TH, Nagle KJ, Lange DJ, Rowland LP. Complications of intravenous immune globulin in neurologic disease. *Neurology* 1996; **47**: 674–677.

23. Kattamis AC, Shankar S, Cohen A. Neurologic complications of treatment of childhood acute immune thrombocytopenic purpura with intravenously administered immunoglobulin G. *J Ped* 1997; **130(2)**: 281–283.

24. Lisak RP. Arthritis associated with circulating immune complexes following administration of intravenous immunoglobulin therapy in a patient with chronic inflammatory demyelinating polyneuropathy. *J Neurol Sci* 1996; **135**: 85–88.

25. Schifferli JA. High-dose intravenous immunoglobulin treatment and renal function. In: Dominioni L, Nydegger UE, eds. *Intravenous Immunoglobulins Today and Tomorrow*. International Congress and Symposium Series 189. London: RSM, 1992, 27–33.

26. Ahsan N, Wiegand LA, Abendroth CS, Manning EC. Acute renal failure following immmunoglobulin therapy. *Am J Nephrol* 1996; **16**: 532–536.

27. Hansen-Schmidt S, Silimon J, Keller F. Osmotic nephrosis due to high-dose immunoglobulin therapy containing sucrose (but not glycine) in a patient with immunoglobulin A nephritis. *Am J Kid Dis* 1996; **28(3)**: 451–453.

28. Ropper AH, Adelman L. Early Guillain–Barré syndrome without inflammation. *Arch Neurol* 1992; **49**: 979–981.

29. Silbert PL, Knezevic WV, Bridge DT. Cerebral infarction complicating intravenous immunoglobulin therapy for polyneuritis cranialis. *Neurology* 1992; **49**: 257–258.

30. Thornton CA, Ballow M. Safety of intravenous immunoglobulin. *Arch Neurol* 1993; **50**: 135–136.

31. Steg RE, Lefkowitz DM. Cerebral infarction following intravenous immunoglobulin

therapy for myasthenia gravis. *Neurology* 1994; **44:** 1180 [clinical/scientific notes].

32. Dalakas MC. High-dose intravenous immunoglobulin and serum viscosity: risk of precipitating thromboembolic events. *Neurology* 1994; **44:** 223–226.

33. Nakamura S, Yoshida T, Ohtake S, Matsuda T. Hemolysis due to high-dose intravenous gammaglobulin treatment for patients with idiopathic thrombocytopenic purpura. *Acta Haemtl* 1986; **76:** 115–118.

34. Comenzo RL, Malachowski ME, Meissner HC et al. Immune hemolysis, disseminated intravascular coagulation, and serum sickness after large doses of immune globulin given intravenously for Kawasaki disease. *J Pediat* 1992; **120:** 926–928.

35. Tamada KI, Kohga M, Masuda H, Hattori K. Hemolytic anemia following high-dose intravenous immunoglobulin administration. *Acta Paedi Japon* 1995; **37(3):** 391–393.

36. Tam DA, Morton LD, Stroncek DF, Leshner RT. Neutropenia in a patient receiving intravenous immune globulin. *J Neuroimm* 1996; **64:** 175–178.

Index

acetylcholine receptor loss, myasthenia gravis 94
acute inflammatory demyelinating polyneuropathy (AIDP) 84, 85, 86
acute motor axonal neuropathy (AMAN) 84, 85, 86
AIDS
   intravenous immunoglobulin treatment
      adults 165–6
      children 163–4
   see also HIV
allergic reactions to intravenous immunoglobulin 155
anaphylactic reactions to intravenous immunoglobulin 155, 161, 188
anti-GM abtibodies, multifocal motor neuropathy 27–9
antibodies
   antiidiotypic 4, 9
   production, suppression by IVIG 4, 6–8

anticholinesterase therapy, myasthenia gravis 95
apoptosis, modulation by IVIG 13
ataxia–telangiectasia 160
Austrian Immunoglobulin in MS (AIMS) trial 104–6, 107, 110
autoantibodies
   neutralization by IVIG 4, 9
   production, suppression by IVIG 4, 6–8
axonal lesions/loss
   chronic inflammatory demyelinating polyneuropathy 58, 60–1
   Guillain–Barré syndrome 84–5
axonal neuropathy
   acute motor 84, 85, 86
   acute motor sensory 85, 86
azathioprine
   inclusion body myositis 68
   Lambert–Eaton myasthenic syndrome 98
   myasthenia gravis 95

B cells, suppression of antibody production by IVIG 4, 6–8
Behçet's disease 115–17
　see also neuro-Behçet syndrome
blood donation 145, 182–3
　individual screening 152
bone marrow transplantation, IVIG treatment 162
burn injuries, IVIG treatment 167

Campylobacter jejuni infection 46
cancer, IVIG treatment 165
CD5-positive cells, inhibition by IVIG 4, 6–8
cell adhesion, inhibition by IVIG 13
cell adhesion molecule, intercellular (ICAM), dermatomyositis, effect of IVIG 75
central nervous system, immune system and 127–8
　epilepsy 128, 129
chlorambucil, neuro-Behçet syndrome 121
chronic inflammatory demyelinating polyneuropathy (CIDP) 34, 43–4
　clinico-pathological findings 58–61
　diagnosis 44–5
　　differential 45–6
　Guillain–Barré syndrome and 47–8
　pathophysiology 46–8
　preceding infections 46–7
　prognostic factors 57–65
　progressive weakness 44–5
　treatment 48–52, 166
　　response to 63
complement
　dermatomyositis, effect of IVIG 75
　neutralization by IVIG 5, 9, 10
conduction block
　anti-GM antibodies and 27
　chronic inflammatory demyelinating polyneuropathy 58–9, 60
　multifocal neuropathies
　　motor 24–7
　　sensory demyelinating 32, 34
corticosteroids
　chronic inflammatory demyelinating polyneuropathy 48, 51, 52
　diabetic lumbosacral radiculoplexoneuropathy 37
　multifocal neuropathies
　　motor 31, 34
　　sensory demyelinating 32, 34
　myasthenia gravis 95
　neuro-Behçet syndrome 121
cranial nerve palsies, diabetic 35
Creutzfeldt–Jakob disease (CJD), contamination of blood donations/IVIG products 145, 182
cyclophosphamide
　inclusion body myositis 68
　multifocal motor neuropathy 31
cyclosporin
　chronic inflammatory demyelinating polyneuropathy 52
　inclusion body myositis 68
　Lambert–Eaton myasthenic syndrome 98
cytokines, TH1/TH2 balance, effects of IVIG 5, 13
cytomegalovirus (CMV) infection in transplant patients, IVIG treatment 162–3

cytotoxicity, antibody-dependent cellular, inhibition by IVIG 9, 10–11
demyelinating polyneuropathy
  acute inflammatory 84, 85, 86
  chronic inflammatory *see* chronic inflammatory demyelinating polyneuropathy
  subacute inflammatory 44
demyelination
  chronic inflammatory demyelinating polyneuropathy 58–9
  Guillain–Barré syndrome 84, 85–6
dermatomyositis 67–9
  intravenous immunoglobulins 68–77
    controlled study 69–72
    mechanism of action 73–7
    role in maintaining response 72
    studies of repeated muscle biopsies and post-IVIG sera 73–7
dexamethasone, chronic inflammatory demyelinating polyneuropathy 52
diabetes mellitus, multifocal neuropathies 20, 21, 35–7
3,4-diaminopyridine (3,4-DAP), Lambert–Eaton myasthenic syndrome 98

epilepsy
  immune system—CNS interactions 128, 129
  malignant, of childhood 128
    immunoglobulin treatment 128–31, 166
    immunological dysfunction in 131–2

Fisher syndrome 85, 86

gangliosides
  antibodies against
    Guillain–Barré syndrome 86
    multifocal motor neuropathy 27–9
  GM1 27
  Guillain–Barré syndrome pathogenesis 86
glatiramer acetate, multiple sclerosis 111
Guillain–Barré syndrome (GBS) 83–91
  electrophysiology 85–6
  immunology 86
  preceding infections 46–7
  progressive weakness 44
  treatment 87–8, 165

headache, intravenous immunoglobulin therapy and 155, 186, 187
hepatitis viruses, blood donations/IVIG products 145, 152, 182
  inactivation/separation procedures 152, 183–4
HIV
  blood donations/IVIG products 145, 152, 182
  inactivation/separation procedures 152
  polymyositis 80–1
  see also AIDS
HLA-B51, Behçet's disease 116, 117
HTLV-1 infection, polymyositis 80–1

idiopathic thrombocytopenic purpura, IVIG treatment 164
immunizations, effect of intravenous immunoglobulins 156

immunodeficiencies, intravenous
    immunoglobulin treatment
  combined immunodeficiencies 160, 161–2
  primary immunodeficiencies 159–62
  secondary immunodeficiencies 162–4,
    165–6
immunoglobulin A (IgA) 138, 139
  selective deficiency 159, 160, 161
immunoglobulin D (IgD) 138–40
immunoglobulin E (IgE) 138, 139
immunoglobulin G (IgG) 138, 139
  catabolism, acceleration after IVIG
    infusion 5, 11
  functions 3, 6
  partial differentiation 7
  structure 2–3, 137
  subclass deficiencies 160, 161
immunoglobulin M (IgM) 138, 139
immunoglobulins 135–6
  intravenous *see* intravenous
    immunoglobulin
  structure and functions 137–40
immunosuppressive drugs
  chronic inflammatory demyelinating
    polyneuropathy 52
  inclusion body myositis 68
  multifocal motor neuropathy 31
  myasthenia gravis 95
  neuro-Behçet syndrome 121
inclusion body myositis 67, 77
  intravenous immunoglobulin treatment
    77–80
infectious neuropathies 21
inflammatory demyelinating polyneuropathy
  acute 84, 85, 86
  chronic *see* chronic inflammatory
    demyelinating polyneuropathy
  subacute 44
inflammatory myopathies 67–8
  intravenous immunoglobulin treatment
    68–81
interferons
  chronic inflammatory demyelinating
    polyneuropathy 52
  multiple sclerosis 111
intravenous immunoglobulin (IVIG)
    135–7
  adverse reactions 154–6, 185–8
    multiple sclerosis patients 110
  AIDS patients, paediatric 163–4
  choice of 156–7, 168–9
  chronic inflammatory demyelinating
    polyneuropathy 49–52, 166
    long-term treatment 50
    mechanism of action 52–3
  clinical uses 159–69
    approved indications 159–65
    experimental indications 166–8
    probably/possibly effective indications
      165–6
  commercially available products 146–51
    comparison 2, 156–8
  dermatomyositis 68–77
    controlled study 69–72
    mechanism of action 73–7
    role in maintaining response 72
    studies of repeated muscle biopsies and
      post-IVIG sera 73–7

diabetic lumbosacral
    radiculoplexoneuropathy 37
epilepsies 130
Guillain–Barré syndrome 87–8, 165
    mechanism of action 52–3
immunomodulatory effects 164–5
inclusion body myositis 77–80
infusion rate 155, 185–6
Lambert–Eaton myasthenic syndrome and
    98–100
mechanisms of action 4–14, 158–9
    chronic inflammatory demyelinating
        polyneuropathy 52–3
    dermatomyositis 73–7
    multifocal neuropathies
        motor 29
        sensory demyelinating 34
    multiple sclerosis 104, 110–12, 167
        adverse effects 110
        Austrian Immunoglobulin in MS study
            104–6, 107, 110
        effects on relapses 106, 108, 109, 111
        monthly MRI and 108–10
    myasthenia gravis 95–7, 167
    neuro-Behçet syndrome 121–2
    pharmacology 144–5
    polymyositis 80
        retroviral-associated 80-1
    production procedure 140, 142–4, 157
        viral inactivation/separation in 152–4,
            183–4
    pyrogen contamination 186
    requirements 140, 141
    safety 136, 181–4

requirements 145, 152–4, 182
tolerability 185–8
transplant recipients 162–3
viral contamination 140, 145, 154, 182
    inactivation/separation procedures
        152–4, 183–4
ischemic neuropathies 21
IVIG *see* intravenous immunoglobulin

Kawasaki's disease, IVIG treatment 164–5

Lambert–Eaton myasthenic syndrome
    (LEMS) 93–4
    diagnosis 98
    pathophysiology 97–8
    treatment 98–100
Lennox–Gastaut syndrome 128, 129
    immunological dysfunction in 131–2
    intravenous immunoglobulin treatment
        130, 131
Lewis–Sumner syndrome 22, 32–4
    treatment 34
lumbosacral radiculoplexoneuropathy (DLR),
    diabetic 36–7
lung cancer, small cell, Lambert–Eaton
    myasthenic syndrome and 97–8, 99

macrophages, effect of IVIG 9, 10-11
magnetic resonance imaging (MRI),
    gadolinium-enhanced, examination of
    effect of IVIG on multiple sclerosis
    108–10
malignancies, IVIG treatment 165
membranolytic attack complex (MAC)

dermatomyositis 68
    effect of IVIG 77
    effect of IVIG 9, 10, 75, 77
meningitis, aseptic, IVIG therapy and 156, 187
methotrexate, inclusion body myositis 68
methylprednisolone, neuro-Behçet syndrome 121
MHC-1, effect of IVIG, dermatomyositis 75, 76
Miller Fisher syndrome 47
mononeuritis multiplex *see* mononeuropathy multiplex
mononeuropathy multiplex 20-2
    causes 20, 21
    confluent 20
motor axonal neuropathy
    acute 84, 85, 86
    acute sensory 85, 86
motor conduction block 24–5
    anti-GM antibodies and 27
    multifocal neuropathies 24–7
mucocutaneous lymph node syndrome, IVIG treatment 164–5
multifocal neuropathies 19–41
    motor neuropathy with persistent conduction block 22–31
        clinical features 23–4
        electrodiagnostic features 24–7
        laboratory features 27–9
        treatment 29–31
    sensorimotor demyelinating (Lewis–Sumner syndrome) 22, 32–4
        diabetic radiculoplexopathies and 35–7
        treatment 34

vasculitic 20, 21, 22
multiple sclerosis 103–4
    intravenous immunoglobulin treatment 104, 110–12, 167
    adverse effects 110
    Austrian Immunoglobulin in MS study 104–6, 107, 110
    effects on relapses 106, 108, 109, 111
    monthly MRI and 108–10
    TH1/TH2 cytokine balance 13
myasthenia gravis 93–4
    diagnosis 94–5
    neonatal 94
    pathophysiology 94
    seronegative 94, 95, 96–7
    treatment 95–7, 166–7
mycophendate, inclusion body myositis 68
myopathies, inflammatory 67–8
    intravenous immunoglobulin treatment 68–81

neonates, low-birthweight, intravenous immunoglobulin treatment 162
neuro-Behçet syndrome 117–21
    extraaxial 119, 120
    parenchymal (intraaxial) 119, 120, 121–2
    treatment 121–2
neuropathy/neuropathies
    acute motor axonal 84, 85, 86
    acute motor sensory axonal 85, 86
    demyelinating 21, 22–34
    infectious 21
    ischemic 21

multifocal *see* multifocal neuropathies
neutrophils, Behçet's disease 116–17

oculomotor neuropathy, diabetic 35
plasmapheresis/plasma exchange
   chronic inflammatory demyelinating
      polyneuropathy 49, 52, 53
   diabetic lumbosacral
      radiculoplexoneuropathy 37
   Guillain–Barré syndrome 87
   Lambert–Eaton myasthenic syndrome 98–9
   multifocal motor neuropathy 31
   myasthenia gravis 95, 96–7
polymyositis 67–8
   intravenous immunoglobulins 80–1
   retroviral-associated 80–1
polyneuropathy
   acute inflammatory demyelinating 84, 85, 86
   chronic inflammatory demyelinating *see*
      chronic inflammatory demyelinating
      polyneuropathy
prednisolone
   Lambert—Eaton myasthenic syndrome 98
   myasthenia gravis 95
prednisone
   along with intravenous immunoglobulins
      dermatomyositis 69, 72
      inclusion body myositis 78–9
   chronic inflammatory demyelinating
      polyneuropathy 48, 51, 52, 53
   inclusion body myositis 68
   neuro-Behçet syndrome 121

radiculoplexopathies, diabetic, multifocal

neuropathies and 35–7
remyelination, IVIG and 13–14
renal side-effects, IVIG therapy 156, 187–8
rheumatic disorders, autoimmune, IVIG
   treatment 167–8

sensory axonal neuropathy, acute motor 85, 86
sepsis, IVIG treatment 167
subacute inflammatory demyelinating
   polyneuropathy (SIDP) 44
superantigens, neutralization by IVIG 4, 12

T cells
   activation, effects of IVIG 4, 11–12
   Behçet's disease 116, 117
thoracic radiculopathy, diabetic 35–6
thrombocytopenic purpura, idiopathic, IVIG
   treatment 164
thymectomy, myasthenia gravis 95
transforming growth factor beta (TGFß),
   inflammatory myopathies, effect of
   IVIG 75, 79
transplant patients, intravenous
   immunoglobulin treatment 162–3

vaccinations, effect of intravenous
   immunoglobulins 156
vasculitic neuropathies, multifocal 20, 21, 22
vasculitis, Behçet's disease 116
venous sinus thrombosis (VST) 119, 120
virus contamination of intravenous
   immunoglobulin 140, 145, 182
   inactivation/separation procedures 152–4,
   183–4

voltage-gated calcium channel (VGCC)
　　antibodies, Lambert–Eaton myasthenic
　　syndrome 97–8
West syndrome 128, 129
　　immunological dysfunction in 131–2
　　intravenous immunoglobulin treatment
　　　130, 131

Wiskott–Aldrich syndrome 160

x-linked antibody deficiency 160
x-linked lymphoproliferative syndrome 160